The
MENOPAUSE
Manual

The
MENOPAUSE
Manual
A woman's guide to the menopause

Wulf. H. Utian

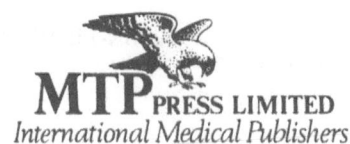

MTP PRESS LIMITED
International Medical Publishers

Published by
MTP Press Limited
Falcon House
LANCASTER

ISBN-13: 978-94-011-7137-3   e-ISBN-13: 978-94-011-7135-9
DOI: 10.1007/978-94-011-7135-9

Acknowledgements

The author gratefully acknowledges permission to reprint material from the following sources:

Hallelujah to Hysterectomy, a poem by a patient of a doctor-friend of the Editor, Obstetrical and Gynecological Survey, April, 1976 (Williams and Wilkins Co., Baltimore).
Oestrogen Therapy, by P. A. van Keep and A. A. Haspels (Excerpta Medica, Amsterdam)

The weight reducing diet under Appendix I is presented with full acknowledgement and thanks to the Dietetic Department and Medical Clinics of Groote Schuur Hospital, Cape Town

To

My parents for teaching me the dictum 'do something properly or not at all'

Moira, Brett and Lara for living with this obsession

Colleagues of the Groote Schuur Hospital Menopause Clinic for their co-operation

My patients for sharing their experiences with me

Contents

8 Contents

Preface

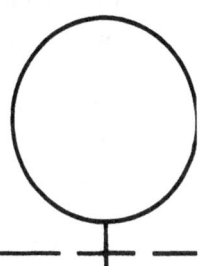

Years of involvement, firsthand experience and research at the Menopause Clinic of the Groote Schuur Hospital, Cape Town, exist as the background to this book. The Clinic itself, however, as one of the first in the world to be established, if not the first, has a story and a lesson of its own to offer, and is therefore deserving of a brief description as the preface to the book.

In 1967, shortly after Christiaan Barnard had completed the historical first human heart transplant at the Groote Schuur Hospital, I happened to be in West Berlin and was invited to visit a major international pharmaceutical firm. A new female hormone was mentioned, and thereby started my interest in the subject. Upon my return to Cape Town, I spent many hours in the large medical school library and completely surveyed the menopause literature to 1967. I was stunned by its general inadequacy and was bitten by a challenge to clarify what menopause really was, and to define the proper place of hormone replacement therapy.

With these objectives in mind, I approached the Chairman of the Department of Gynecology at the University of Cape Town, Professor Dennis Davey, and spelled out my plans for a menopause clinic. Ten years previously I might have been thrown out of the office for presenting a crackpot idea. But Doctor Davey was a scientist at heart and received the idea with enthusiasm, and in the 10 years following his decision maintained the same positive support for me as well as the Clinic. My own career in menopause research therefore parallels that of the Clinic.

The name of the Clinic changed from the Menopause Clinic to the Femininity Clinic and finally to the Mature Women's Clinic and was inundated with requests for appointments. Originally established as a research centre, its contributions in this respect have been considerable. A close understanding of the problems confronting hundreds of women gave rare insight and perspective. This perspective and the ideas it produced are presented in Chapter 13.

The concept of a Menopause Clinic, by whatever title, is of extreme value and deserves a place in all large hospitals and medical centres. Let me explain:

1. The centre functions as a 'well-woman' clinic, designed to attract women from age 45 onward (or earlier with premature menopause). An opportunity is provided for participants to receive medical checkups, be screened for breast cancer, high blood pressure, diabetes, etc.
2. All patients with menopausal problems are seen by one group of doctors and involved personnel who are highly experienced in this area.
3. Follow up therapy is far more efficiently controlled and the patient herself is better able to get to know and become involved with one doctor or group of doctors.
4. The centre can develop a research function. This does not imply that the patient is used as an experimental model, but a continuous search after new knowledge is of vital concern to each woman who uses the facilities of the clinic.
5. The clinic becomes a welcoming, friendly place to the patients enrolled, much like a club. The clinic staff support each other and in doing so, create a highly attractive environment for the patient who may feel alone and in need of a chat.

Evidence for the above statement was that I would occasionally arrive late at the clinic for consultations. If I offered apologies to the women who were waiting, these were usually brushed away with the comment 'we were only too pleased to wait; we have so much in common to discuss'. Obviously there had to be a lesson in this. This was to create groups of women with similar interests and let them support each other, but still have available either an interested physician or a menopause clinic on which to call when necessary. Thus began the concept of a Menopause Support Group.

The hope for the future is that centres such as these will become readily available to those women who may need them. Hopefully by the end of this book you will be so well informed that the decision to look for such a centre would be of your own choosing, not because of lack of information.

1 Introduction

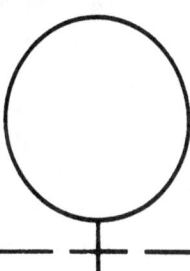

The need to know

A friend of mine complained recently that the press and magazines were full of articles about estrogens and menopause, but that the more she read the less she knew or understood. This seemed most unfortunate as the subject is one of such direct importance to every woman.

The need was for a straightforward explanatory book. But how does one provide all the information on an authoritative basis and still keep it easy to read? What format to use? A pleasant simple to read story book that once read could be discarded; or a detailed reference book to grace the bookshelf and that may never be read?

This is the Menopause Manual. As a story and reference book combined, it is meant to be read initially like a novel and then kept for constant reference whenever the need arises. Only remember that this story book has a difference. It is true to life and the main character is you. Moreover the stakes are high – a happy and effective life on the one hand, or possible ignorance, misery and discontent on the other.

Within these pages you will find all the facts about menopause. New ideas for the development of a different and exciting life style after menopause will be presented. Hopefully you will read the facts and heed the advice.

One point bears emphasis. Although this is a complete guide to menopause it is not a hormonal do-it-yourself kit. In other words, where hormones and medical care are necessary, don't try any shortcuts. See your doctor. The big difference is that when you do so, you will be fully informed and able to discuss things on a one-to-one basis.

The popular image of menopause is as much a frame of mind as a state of bodily change. There are numerous descriptions and misconceptions as to what the 'change of life' is really all about. Few of these stories match each other, except that none ever paint a pretty picture of what to expect.

Little wonder that many a woman approaches this significant event in her life with nothing short of dread, anxiety and fear. In desperation she is likely to turn for guidance to friends or family, to women's magazines or the lay medical press. Where does this all get her? She simply gets confused – a confusion that aggravates the distorted image she may have of life and where it is taking her.

'There is nothing to it', says one friend, but 'it is the change of life and beginning of old age', says another. 'My sex life ended and my husband left me', confides her next door neighbour, while her aunt warns: 'take life easy or you will break a bone'. 'Menopause is a galloping catastrophe' states one physician but hurries on to add that with hormone therapy 'you will be much more pleasant to live with and will not become dull and unattractive'. 'You must be crazy to allow a male chauvinist gynecologist to give you hormones. Don't you know they cause cancer?' shouts her daughter. And so it goes on with confusion, more indecision and greater emotional stress the escalating result.

Whose fault is this distorted idea of menopause? Probably ignorance, aided and abetted by societal attitudes, fallacies and misconceptions. The situation, moreover, has often been traded upon by groups as disparate as manufacturers of teen-age fashions, the pharmaceutical industry, sports goods producers and operators of health farms. Their message inevitably perpetuates the myth that young is beautiful and that old is ugly.

Did you know: that some women look forward to menopause? that the average European female has less anxiety about menopause and ageing than her American sister? that stresses and strains are placed on many people by the so-called 'youth-culture'? Do you expect a change in your sex life as inevitable? Are you considering taking hormones but not really sure what to do? Do you in fact know what menopause or climacteric or hormones really are?

This book provides the answers to these questions and many more. Written expressly for the concerned woman, it should be read by men too. They need some insight into the problems of menopause, as well as some understanding of the women with whom they associate. Men should know that male menopause is as real an entity as the female counterpart and many principles developed in this book could well apply to them.

The purpose is to make facts understandable, so the language will be simple. Do not be misled by this as the information is authentic nonetheless. No attempt is made to bore you with every source of information; if you feel inspired to read in greater depth, the suggested list of references at the end of the book will show you the way.

Medical research is accelerating at a furious pace. Any medically orientated book could be criticized for being out of date before it is even published. Such criticism is only true about the leading edge of research. But an understanding of the basic facts, that is the ABC, is necessary before new aspects of research can be appreciated. This book should provide the average person with these basic building blocks. Thereafter each new piece of information can be better measured and new and real advances truly recognized.

Menopause is much more than hormones. Other aspects too, like the way you live your life, sexual activity and the attitudes of society will be considered. The positive concept to be given for a new lifestyle after menopause is based on straightforward principles that really work.

Very little in life that is genuinely worthwhile comes easy. This book is no more than a guide or practical handbook, much the equivalent of a television or new car instruction manual. The difference is that the appliance described is you yourself. It needs to be understood. You will then be better able to judge your own needs after the menopause, hormonal and other, and 'change of life' can truly be made to mean 'change for the better'.

2 Historical perspective

A look at yesterday to help you understand today and live with tomorrow

The finalization of menstruation has been recorded from biblical times. As far back as 1777 efforts were made to explain the reason for the discontinuance of the menstrual cycle. Many of these attempts were no more than guesses, some of them entirely false. The general idea offered by these early pioneers in the field of menstrual function was that the blood stopped flowing to the womb, that cessation of the function meant the impress of age was on a woman's face, or that her genital organs were sealed with sterility.

The attitudes were also totally negative. Statements were made that it was ridiculous for her to think about sexual enjoyment, that her charms were gone forever, even that she ceased to be part of the human species.

As for the treatments attempted, various ideas were put forth regarding methods to decrease the incidence of hot flushes and the use of 'half a pint of old, clear London porter or a glass of Rhenish wine' was offered as one antidote. One physician had the gall to write that all would be well if the bowels were kept open.

Just how long did these attitudes persist? It may surprise you that a look at the medical literature as recent as 1967 indicated that some physicians felt that the termination of the reproductive phase in a woman's life was an event destined to throw her into considerable turmoil or would make her a negative, harmless creature. It was called a 'tragedy' and, in more than one reference, considered to actually be a 'catastrophe' which, somehow, the female must muddle through and still make an attempt to be attractive, mentally alert and lead a productive life.

What is the true picture? Before going into the 'today' concept of menstrual cessation, let us look briefly into the field of so-called hormone or estrogen replacement treatment after menopause. A recent development? Not exactly.

GLANDULAR OR OVARIAN TREATMENT

Glandular therapy was a very ancient form of treatment. The Egyptians, Greeks and Romans all prescribed various cures for impotence, some as bizarre as swallowing the testis of an ass. In 1888 one physician reported he was 'rejuvenating' himself by injections of testicular juice, and claimed he could do the same for his wife.

At the close of the nineteenth century, ovarian therapy was limited to the use of such things as powdered ovaries and powdered ovarian tablets. These substances were used for the treatment of painful periods, obesity and physiological or surgical menopause.

As you know, such 'miracle' health cures are still in our society. Monkey gland transplants occasionally make news as well as the names of the exclusive clinics tucked away in exotic mountain resort areas of Central Europe which offer secret treatments against ageing with the only limiting factors for their claims being the size of the bank balance or the gullibility of the prospective clients.

THE DEVELOPMENT OF THE FEMALE HORMONES

Early investigators became aware of 'internal secretions' way back in 1775.

It was not until the present century that the modern understanding of how the ovaries function started to take shape. This was helped by discoveries such as that made by Doctors Stockard and Papanicolaou in 1917 that examination of vaginal cells under the microscope showed changes relating directly to the stage of the egg or hormone-producing cycle. This work was also to be the beginning of what we know today as the Pap smear.

Later came the development of tests for measurements of the

levels of female hormones. Not long after, the discovery was made of the actual female hormones oestrone, oestriol and oestradiole. These were initially extracted from human pregnancy urine. Later their complex chemical structure was found out. A word on the spelling of these substances. The female hormones had names derived from oestrus or heat in animals. The spelling has been abbreviated to estrus without the o and this is gradually becoming internationally accepted.

Soon these new hormones were to be made available to doctors for clinical use.

THE WONDER DRUG?

With the advent of estrogen, papers began to be published in medical journals extolling its virtues. Books were written on the subject. One of them, *Feminine Forever* written in 1965 by Doctor Robert A. Wilson, represents a landmark in the written history of menopause despite the many failings that it had. It placed the subject directly in the spotlight of public attention and in the hands of the media, thereby succeeding in firing excessive expectations and literally opening the floodgates of patient demand.

This, of course, presented a grave problem. Women of the ages to be interested in menopause directly regarding themselves or others, looked to estrogen as the answer to all problems. But much research still had to be done in this field. What were the risks involved in its use? What were the actual benefits? Were there any side-effects? If so, what were they and how could they be avoided or treated? Obviously a closer, longer look was needed to define the claims for the puberty-to-the-grave estrogens.

Deficiencies in the original methods of treatment were uncovered. Just one example of the deficiencies was that the ovaries produce different hormones at different times of the cycle. The estrogen replacement, in the way it was being given, did not match up to this behaviour of mother nature.

Many questions remained to be answered. Efforts were started around the world to define the word 'climacteric' (see page 25). What are the associated effects? What are the risks? Are they due to loss of hormones? What effects are not related to hormones? What is the best treatment?

A large amount of work has been done and an increasing volume is being done in many leading hospitals and clinics throughout the world. The expansion of recent knowledge has been nothing short of electrifying. The postmenopause is becoming more and more an area for study by the physician, the clinical chemist, the pharmaceutical industry and pathologists. More on the subject of estrogens relating to you will be explained later on in the book.

The enormous publicity devoted to the debate about estrogen treatment after the menopause had therefore succeeded in stirring up a lot of action. The large number of women requiring some sort of assistance became evident and the need for specific forms of supportive therapy was highlighted. Women could now voice their concerns without being put off with a comment from their husband or a physician that 'it's all in your mind'. Women were made aware of the existence of Hormone Replacement Therapy and the choice they could now have regarding the menopause. Doctors have been alerted to the possible treatments and also the need for treatment. A woman may, with dignity, decide she needs medical help to get her through this period in her life and no longer need to feel embarrassment when she requests this help.

There is much yet to be done, but all in all, a new enlightened era has dawned.

3 Changing populations and vital statistics

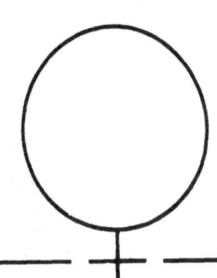

The gradual demise of the 'youth culture' and the impact of ageing populations

For several years it appeared as if the onset of menopause was coming on at an older and older age. Indeed with the possibility of a decreasing age of menarche and an increasing age of menopause, it looked as if modern woman was becoming more fertile by expanding her reproductive years. But this is not so. The median age at natural menopause is 50.8 years. There is no conclusive evidence of an increase in age at menopause over the last century.

One fact does stand out. No female need fear that she stands alone as she approaches menopause. There has been a real increase in the actual number of women reaching and living well beyond this time. Newspaper headlines have warned: NEW POPULATION TRENDS TRANSFORMING U.S. These trends really do exist. They are occurring throughout the developed world and have far reaching implications for the future. Let us take a brief look at what is happening to the world and the human population on it.

Some countries have a high birth rate resulting in a large population of young people. These are usually the underdeveloped countries. Disease rates are invariably higher and this results in fewer people living to old age.

Some countries have a low growth rate. These are inevitably highly developed countries where zero population growth has become a reality. Here we would see many more old people compared to relatively fewer young people. That is, there are less babies, and with better health services there are more people living to an older age.

An example of a high birth rate country is Mexico, and Sweden is typical of a country with a low birth rate. The 1970 population of the United States fell somewhere between the high rate of growth of Mexico and the low rate of growth of Sweden. In other words the birth rate is falling and the real number of older people is increasing.

There has been another change as well. In 1900 the median age of people in the United States was 22.9 years. By 1950 it was 30.2. It is projected to be 34.8 at the turn of the century and 37.3 by the year 2030. This means that the average age of the population is gradually increasing. The increased number of people living to an old age can be more easily imagined if you realise that 1 in 10 of the population today is aged over 65. By 2030 this figure will be 1 in 6. At present some 11 per cent of all women in Western Europe are aged between 45 and 55 years.

Consider what all this means in terms of changes in housing requirements, land use, recreational facilities, medical care, retirement and health insurance and so forth. School enrolments will drop and clothing fashions will change. Social security taxation will alter in that a greater burden will have to be carried by a smaller population.

Not everyone is in full agreement as to what will really happen. Alfred Sauvy, a French demographer, envisages an ageing society as one 'that would slide towards inevitable decadence, like a tree with too much foliage for there to be any young growth'. He foresees a 'population of old people ruminating over old ideas in old houses'. Others concede that the transition to an older society may have painful dislocations, but they do not believe that the ultimate effect will be damaging.

We can now examine the situation a little more closely for the postmenopausal woman.

There is unequivocal evidence that the population of postmenopausal women over the age of 50 has changed significantly during the course of the past century. The life expectation for a woman born during the time of the Roman Empire was about 29 years. During the late mediaeval period this increased to 33 years. By 1841, in England and Wales, the average female life expectancy had reached 42 years. A dramatic change developed during the late nineteenth and early twentieth centuries and the expectation of life at birth had increased to 74.9 years by 1970. This represents an increase of 68 per cent over the past century.

But looking at how many years a woman was likely to live from birth onwards can be very misleading. Most women in the early days died from complications in childbirth or the effects of various epidemics, and fewer were left to live into old age. It is more correct to check the number of years a woman can expect to live after the age of 50. This has in fact increased from 20.6 years to 28.3 years over the last one hundred years, and represents an increase of only 7.7 years or 37 per cent. Thus more women have been reaching the increased age, and the overall increase in life expectancy after menopause is only increasing at a slow rate. Nonetheless, the average woman today can expect to live at least one third of her life in the postmenopausal phase.

The life expectancy of the male has not matched that of the female. This creates an increasing proportion of widowed or single women. Unless the death rate of men is drastically cut, the gap in lifespan between men and women is likely to widen, even though both will live longer. The half-jokingly made suggestion that bigamy be legalised for elderly men hardly provides an answer to the problem. Indeed it is more likely to make it worse.

The quantity of postmenopausal life expectancy has thus been defined. The next step is to look at the quality of this time of life. In this respect the actual symptoms and their severity vary in different educational, social and cultural groups and the background to this will become obvious in the next chapter.

4 The social, cultural and emotional aspects

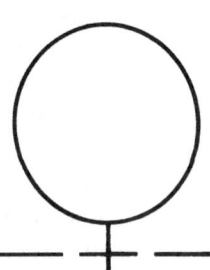

How the attitudes of others can affect your own response to menopause

The climacteric syndrome is complex and not merely a matter of hormones.

The development of symptoms during the climacteric is referred to as the climacteric syndrome. These symptoms are severe enough to cause about 10 to 15 per cent of the women so affected to seek medical advice. For reasons that will become clear, this figure varies considerably from country to country.

Just as the proportion of women seeking medical assistance varies, so does the actual type of symptom vary as well. This is because there are several possible mechanisms that can produce these symptoms. Moreover, there is a strong interaction between the different mechanisms. In this chapter we will outline the mechanisms and discuss some of them. The others will be dealt with in turn later in the book.

The background mechanisms that produce symptoms at menopause are:

1. The concurrent ageing process and coincidental diseases
2. Decrease of hormones from the ovary
3. Social and cultural factors – the impact of the environment
4. Psychological factors – the nature of the personality.

Our present purpose is to look at the social, cultural and psychological components.

Certain social and cultural factors can be shown to have positive effects in reducing climacteric problems. On the other hand, adverse circumstances are present in some socio-cultural environments and these add to climacteric syndrome related problems. Let me offer some concrete examples to explain the above more clearly.

Put into simple terms, some societies reward women for having reached menopause or the end of the fertile period, while others in effect actually punish them.

Look at the situation with some African tribes. The women after menopause graduate from being 'bearers of children and drawers of water' to full tribal equality. They can sit in on the tribal council and participate in full decision making, and in effect become a fully-fledged member of the 'tribal parliament'. Little wonder, menopause for these women is looked forward to as a positive experience.

A similar situation has been described for certain Arab women for whom the end of the fertile period brings positive changes in their lives.

Another striking illustration of this cultural attitude is shown with women of the Rahjput classes in India. They experience few symptoms and look forward to menopause because they emerge from Purdah at the end of their childbearing years. They acquire higher status because they are no longer 'contaminated' by menstrual blood. In this instance, the attitude to menopause may be positive, but the one to menstruation is negative.

On the opposite extreme, in most Western societies there is a strong emphasis on the 'youth culture'. Being young and beautiful becomes a matter of prime concern. Cosmetics, mode of dress and the correct youthful image become important. The popularity of plastic surgery has been described as a reflection of the punitive attitude toward the menopause and ageing. Women from such societies see nothing positive about menopause other than a reminder that they are no longer young.

Many other stresses and strains develop around the age of menopause. Thus the average woman of 50 finds her social status to have changed. It is most likely that she will lose one or both parents at that time. In most instances her children will leave home, either for college or because of marriage. She may become a mother-in-law or a grandmother or both. It is possible that her husband may become ill.

These are all social components but liable to produce psychological stresses dependent on the basic character of the woman affected.

Modern evaluation of the impact of ageing on menopause has shown one reassuring feature. It does not come on as the sudden catastrophe so popularly described. Doctor Gertrude Krüskemper, working in Dusseldorf, has shown that personality profiles are remarkably constant and this suggests that the impact of the climacteric on a woman's personality is in no way dramatic.

Several studies have shown that important alternate roles at the time of menopause, for example a profession, or being the sole wage earner, lessen the symptom profile of the climacteric. Similarly patient education may have a positive effect in this respect.

The lessons to be learned from the above observations are important. It is misleading to consider the climacteric phase as being purely a biological phenomenon, that is as being simply due to a lack of hormones. Social and cultural behaviour patterns directly contribute to the image of menopause.

Large scale educational programmes are necessary to explain positive attitudes, and hence improve this incorrect image. By the same measure it appears that education of women in their early 40's can help them live through the climacteric with minimal problems.

In all these instances then the one necessary step appears to be education. But more can be accomplished than by just education about what not to expect. An aggressive positive attitude to life itself and where it is taking you is necessary. For the moment we will continue with the education process directed at you the reader; the new attitude to your life style itself will be developed later in the book.

5 Female structure and function

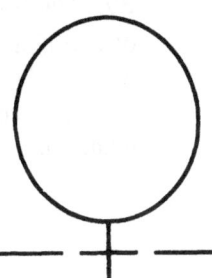

The what, where and why – or the organs and how they work

ANATOMY: The science of the structure of the animal body
PHYSIOLOGY: The science which treats of the functions of the
  living organism and its parts
                              Dorlands Illustrated Medical Dictionary
                              (24th Edition)

This chapter represents the technical section of this book. Some readers may not like the word technical and feel inclined to put the book aside because they expect to find it heavy going. Fight the impulse. The language is simple and even scanning this section will add to your knowledge. The majority will find this chapter provides an exciting glimpse into the unique background of the perpetuation of life itself.

The human body is an exquisite mechanism. Every single function inevitably involves many other parts and processes. This is true in part for a motorcar or a TV set. But they cannot control themselves, and therein lies the difference.

To understand how something works, you first need to know about each of its parts. In medicine the description of the parts is called anatomy and how they work is termed physiology. We are about to take a brief look at both.

THE PARTS – ANATOMY

Early gynaecologists often regarded their speciality as starting at the belly button and ending at the top of the thighs. That was a way of avoiding what they really knew very little about. Inevitably it became clear that the female monthly cycle was under the control of certain centres in the brain. You too should know about these higher brain centres, and that is where we will start.

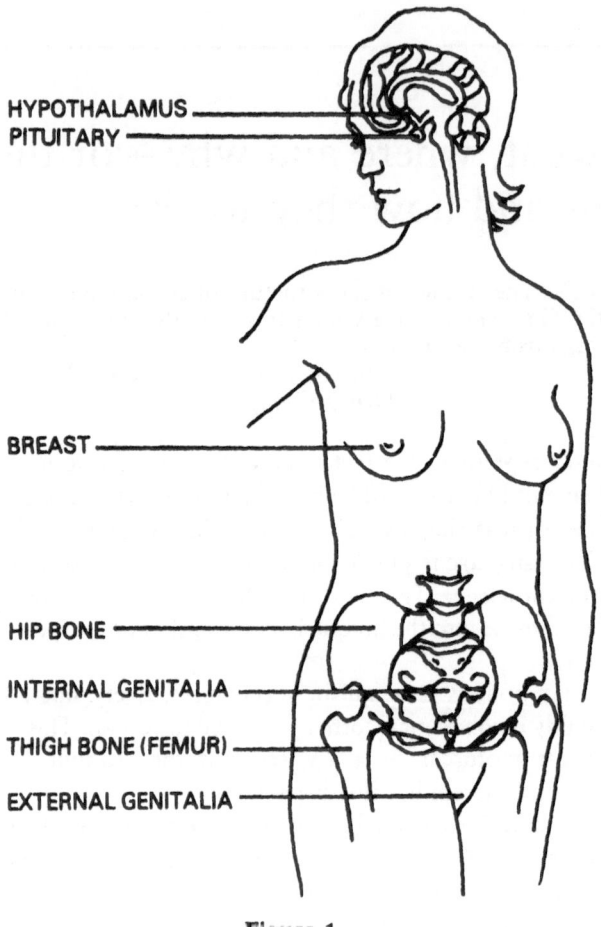

HYPOTHALAMUS
PITUITARY

BREAST

HIP BONE

INTERNAL GENITALIA

THIGH BONE (FEMUR)

EXTERNAL GENITALIA

Figure 1

The position of the organs about to be described are indicated in Figure 1. This sketch, as with all the other illustrations, is simplified to prove a point and makes no pretence at anatomical perfection.

The author has done these illustrations himself to help as a visual guide along the way.

Hypothalamus

Virtually in the middle of the skull lies an organ with an impossible sounding name. The *hypothalamus* is to the human body the equivalent of what the ground control co-ordinating centre is to moon rockets and space flight. It is an actual part of the lower surface of the brain and has a shape resembling a funnel.

Impulses or messages from the outside senses like sight, smell, hearing, taste and touch are directed eventually to the hypothalamus (Figure 2), and this central area of the brain is connected to virtually

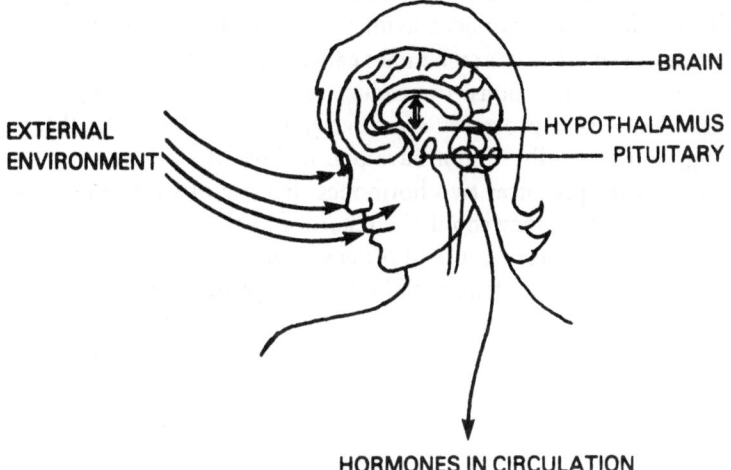

EXTERNAL ENVIRONMENT

BRAIN

HYPOTHALAMUS

PITUITARY

HORMONES IN CIRCULATION

Figure 2

all the other areas of the brain. The hypothalamus has the uncanny ability to co-ordinate much of this information.

The hypothalamus makes a messenger called a *hormone*. Hormones are chemicals released into the blood by any of the specialized glands in the body called *endocrine glands*. The hypothalamic hormone that is of importance to our understanding of the female monthly cycle is called *gonadotropin releasing hormone* (abbreviated to GRH). Do not be put off by the name; we will explain it later.

Pituitary gland

Directly beneath the hypothalamus in a boney cave in the base of the skull lies the pea-sized structure called the *pituitary gland*. It is also an endocrine gland which means that it, too, can make hormones. There are two that are of interest to us. Together they are usually called the *gonadotropins* and the reason will soon become clear. The names of the individual gonadotropins are: *follicle stimulating hormone* (FSH) and *luteinizing hormone* (LH).

Once again, do not be bothered by the fancy names. They will soon become self-explanatory.

Ovary

The third endocrine gland that needs introduction, even though like all the others you have been living with it all your life, is the *ovary*, or *female gonad* as it is sometimes called. There are two ovaries and they have two functions: to produce sex hormones and to produce eggs. These two processes are directly inter-related. Like the old song, you generally cannot have one without the other.

The ovary produces two hormones that are of such importance to our story that they should be regarded as the central characters. Their names are *estrogen* and *progesterone*.

Before birth of the female child there are probably several million eggs in the ovaries, but for reasons not known, this number reduces and at birth there are only about 500 000 eggs remaining. Unlike the male who is able to produce new spermatazoa for the rest of his life, the fem. ε ovary continues to lose eggs until the supply is virtually exhausted at the menopause. But more of this later.

If an ovary is cut in half numerous little structures become visible on the cut surface. What you see is actually dependent upon the age of the female and, if she is of child-bearing age, the stage of the monthly cycle. All the possibilities are shown in Figure 3.
In summary therefore:

1. The ovary produces eggs and hormones.
2. The names of the female sex hormones are *estrogen* and *progesterone*.
3. The structure that produces the egg and sex hormones within the ovary has a different appearance as it develops during the monthly cycle.

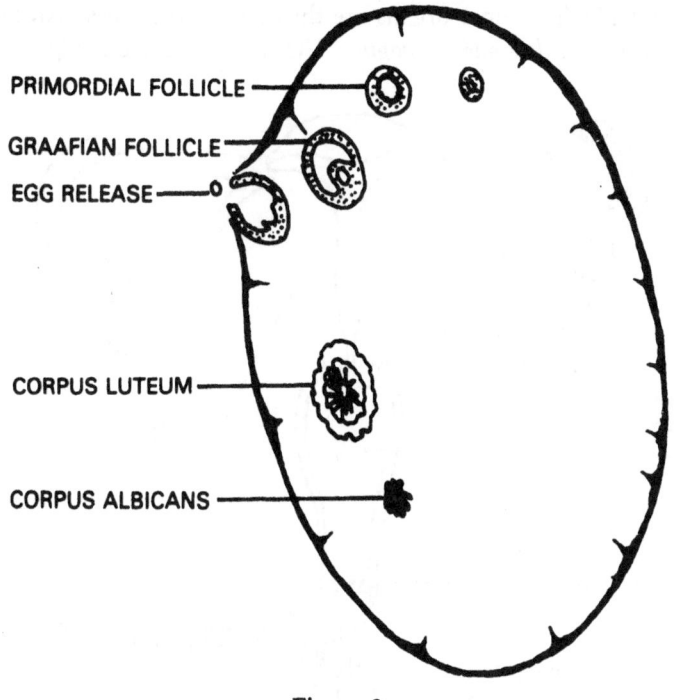

PRIMORDIAL FOLLICLE

GRAAFIAN FOLLICLE

EGG RELEASE

CORPUS LUTEUM

CORPUS ALBICANS

Figure 3

Primordial follicle   This is the early egg surrounded b issue cells.
Graafian follicle   This produces *estrogen* in the first 2 weeks of the
monthly cycle and releases the egg after that.
Corpus luteum   This is a yellow body or bump which produces
estrogen and *progesterone* after the egg has been released. It ages
and shrivels into a *corpus albicans*.
Corpus albicans   This is a small, dense, white structure without
any function.

You probably will have noticed that each of these little
structures forms from the one before it on the list. Once again the
names are not the matters of importance. But our two characters
estrogen and *progesterone* are. We will meet them again later.

Other sex organs

The female sex organs are divided into structures on the inside and the outside. The inner organs are the *ovaries*, the *uterus* (womb), the *fallopian tubes* and the *vagina*. They are illustrated in Figure 4.

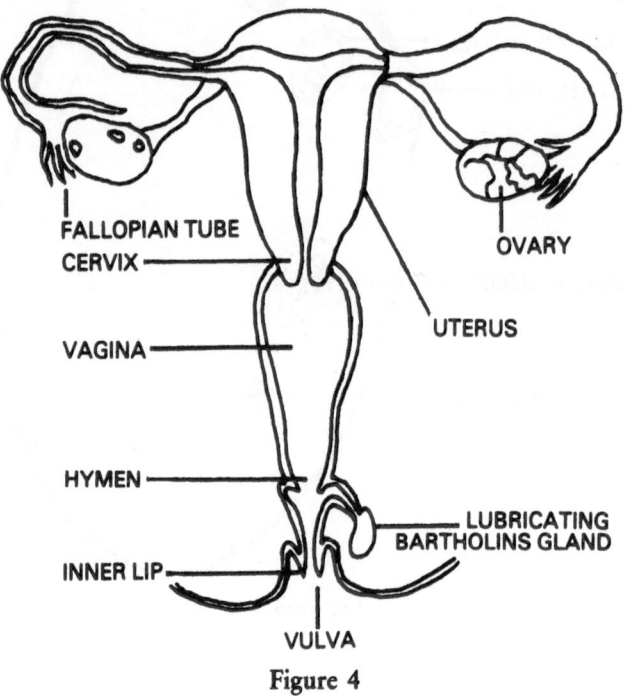

Figure 4

The outer area of the genitalia and vagina, called the *vulva*, has a major sex function. Each of the separate parts are shown in Figure 5.

Other organs found in the pelvis

Apart from the sex organs other organs are found in the pelvis. These are more easily understood if we look at a diagram of the pelvis cut in cross section down the centre of the body, as in Figure 6.

The neighbours of the sex organs are the *bladder*, which lies in front of the uterus, and the *urethra* (tube leading from the bladder to the exterior), which lies in front of the vagina. The *bowel* lies behind the uterus and the *rectum* and *anus* (opening of the bowel to the exterior) lie behind the vagina.

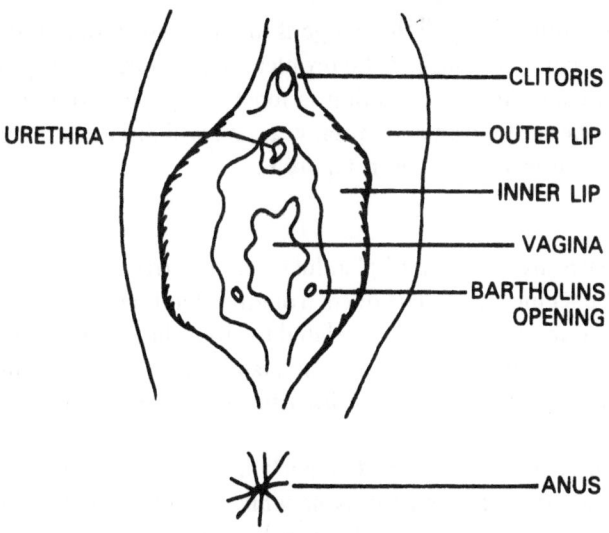

Figure 5

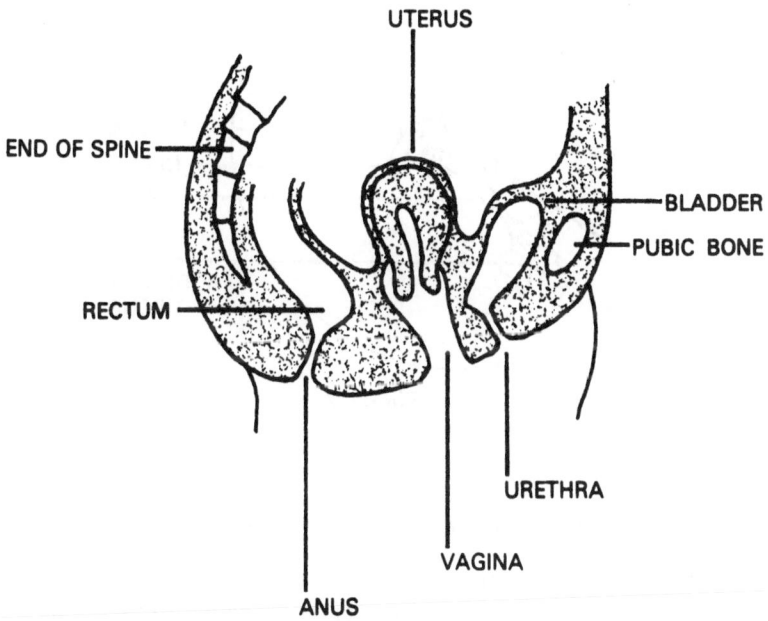

Figure 6

The relationship of all these organs to the vagina is of importance when we come to consider the problem of *prolapse* or drop of the pelvic organs. As this condition is most likely to become bothersome in the early postmenopausal years we will discuss it later. The normal anatomy is shown in Figure 6.

Breasts

The breasts are made up of glandular tissue surrounded by fat as a form of packing tissue. The ducts from the glands end in the nipple. The function of breasts is not related to size. The important fact to remember about breasts is that the glands can react to hormones and also that they are the site for cancer when it develops in the breast.

Fibrous bands known as Cooper's ligaments run through the breast and attach to the firm tissue which lies like a sheet covering the muscle of the chest wall. Stretch of these bands is said to account for breast hang, or 'Cooper's droop'. The anatomy is shown in Figures 7 and 8.

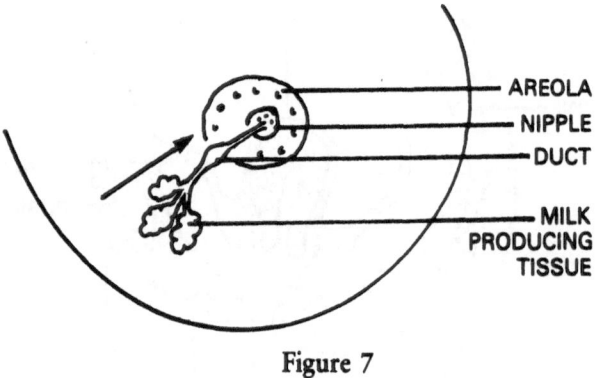

AREOLA
NIPPLE
DUCT
MILK PRODUCING TISSUE

Figure 7

HOW THE PARTS WORK – PHYSIOLOGY

Hopefully you have managed to reach this point relatively painlessly. The brief description of the parts probably prompts questions like what do they do, or how do they work? The answers will now be provided for these questions.

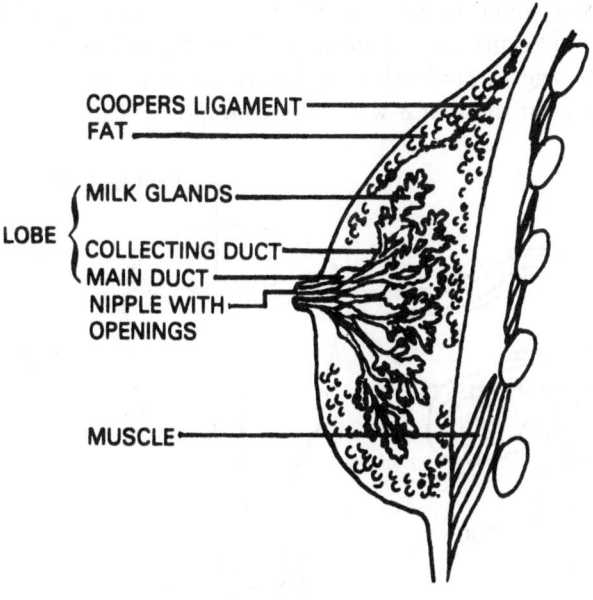

COOPERS LIGAMENT
FAT
MILK GLANDS
LOBE {
COLLECTING DUCT
MAIN DUCT
NIPPLE WITH
OPENINGS
MUSCLE

Figure 8

The events during life over which you have no control

Let us first take a down to earth look at those events in life which are inevitable. They are summarized in Figure 9.

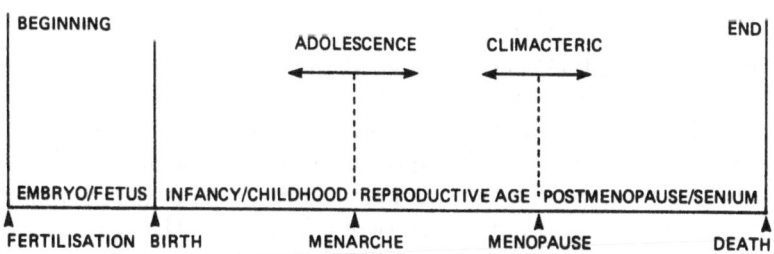

BEGINNING   ADOLESCENCE   CLIMACTERIC   END

EMBRYO/FETUS | INFANCY/CHILDHOOD | REPRODUCTIVE AGE | POSTMENOPAUSE/SENIUM

FERTILISATION BIRTH   MENARCHE   MENOPAUSE   DEATH

Figure 9. Schematic diagram of the significant phases and events in the human life cycle

Without entering into the debate on the beginnings of life, an individual begins with fertilization, that is the joining of the sperm and the egg. Examination of Figure 10 will show where this happens. For the first 8 weeks the conceptus is called the *embryo*

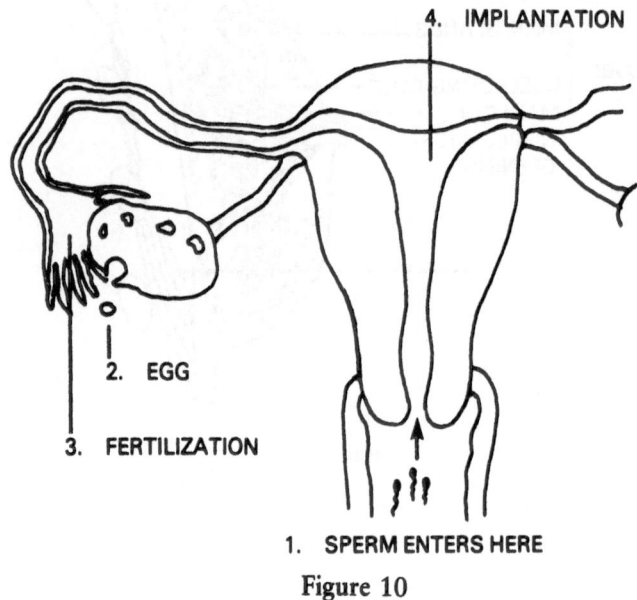

Figure 10

because it is still forming organs like heart and lungs. After that it becomes the *fetus*, and growth occurs over the rest of the pregnancy.

Birth itself is a landmark, the visible beginning of the human life cycle. Not one of us knows what fate has in store for us. But like day follows night, certain events are inevitable. Look back to Figure 9 and these events are immediately obvious.

Following *birth* the baby in growing proceeds through *infancy* and *childhood*. Late childhood or the 'teens' will be marked by a distinct event, the first menstrual period or *menarche,* and the time around this event is called *puberty* or *adolescence.* This marks the entrance into the *reproductive age* of the female and will continue until the final menstrual period or *menopause.* The time-related events around the menopause are usually collectively named the *climacteric* and is followed by a period of several years called the *postmenopause*. The latter gradually merges into the *senium* or old age, only to eventually and inevitably be terminated by *death*.

Some of the above names deserve a little extra comment.

Climacteric The change from the reproductive stage of life to the non-reproductive stage usually happens between 45 and 55 years of age, and means no more and no less than this.

Menopause This indicates the *final menstrual period* and occurs during the climacteric. It occurs on average at 51 years of age, and represents one of life's most significant landmarks, indicating two thirds down, one third to go and make the most of it.

Climacteric syndrome A syndrome in medical language is a group of symptoms. The climacteric is not always associated with symptoms, but if they occur we call it the climacteric syndrome.

Senium Gradually the postmenopausal woman will age physically and emotionally and will enter the senium or old age. The adage that you are as old as you feel holds much truth, but the inevitable end of the senium is death.

The above events are inevitable, but some of the features can be modified by advances in medical science supported by a direct effort on the part of yourself. Read on and you will see what I mean.

The production of hormones during the reproductive age

The reproductive cycle, also called the menstrual or ovulatory cycle, is the key to re-creation itself. I will attempt to explain it in the most simple way. Make use of the diagrams as you read the text.

Each menstrual or egg producing cycle commences with the first day of the period (Day 1). At that point there is very little hormone around. Start at the beginning of Figure 11:

Low levels of hormones remind the hypothalamus that it is time for another attempt at pregnancy with a new egg producing cycle. The hypothalamus sends a burst of its hormone messenger GRH to the pituitary gland and stimulates release of *follicle stimulating hormone* (FSH). FSH does just that. It travels to the ovary and stimulates a Graafian follicle to grow and to pour *estrogen* into the blood stream. The gradual progression of the cycle through Days 7 to 14 is shown in Figure 12 and described below.

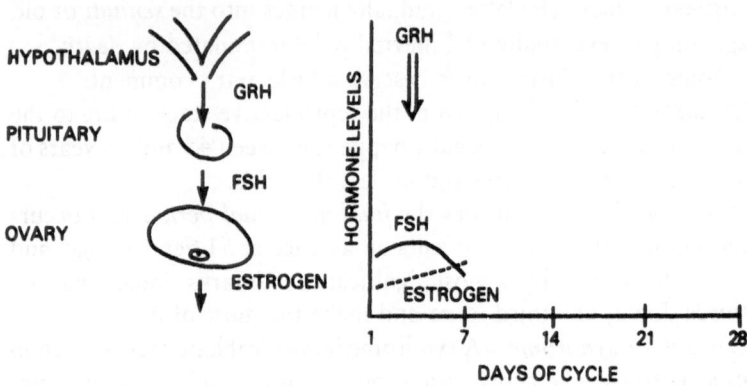

Figure 11

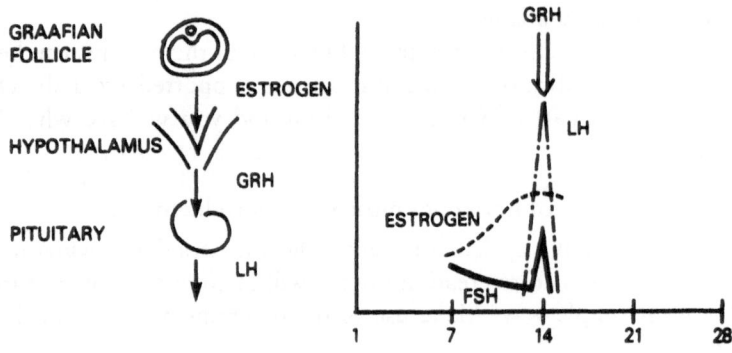

Figure 12

Estrogen production peaks at Day 14, the middle of the cycle. The hypothalamus interprets this message as the good news indicating that the follicle is ripe and ready to free the egg. Another GRH messenger rushes to the pituitary gland and sends *luteinizing hormone* to the ovary because of its powers in releasing the egg.

Following loss of the egg the Graafian follicle changes into the yellow corpus luteum, and this is able to make estrogen and progesterone for nearly 14 days without any reminders from headquarters.

Eventually the corpus luteum shrivels into the corpus albicans and stops producing hormones. These levels will become so low that space control centre in the hypothalamus will be prompted to start the whole cycle off again.

The changes discussed above are illustrated in Figure 13.

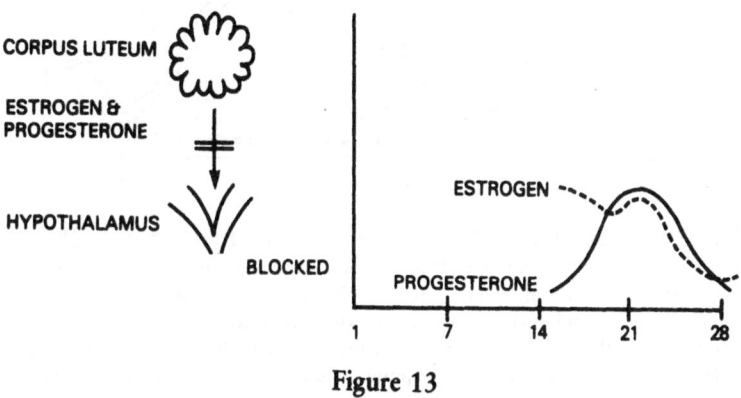

Figure 13

In summary therefore the reproductive cycle is best depicted as in Figure 14.

The changes in the amounts of hormone after menopause

Having completed that section you may be heaving a sigh of relief, and ask what has all that to do with menopause anyway? In fact, a lot. It results in estrogen and progesterone production. This runs out after menopause.

Remember the ovary is presented before birth with its total complement of eggs and no new ones will ever be formed again. After some 35 years of regular menstrual cycles, interrupted only by any pregnancies that may have occurred, the ovary runs out of its supply of eggs, and the following is what happens to the hormones.

Headquarters works overtime producing large amounts of GRH and FSH and LH but the poor old ovary is exhausted and cannot

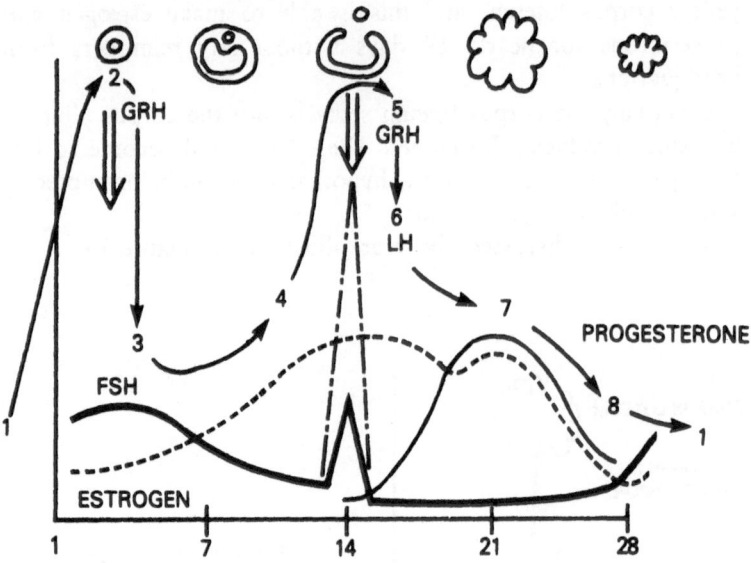

Figure 14. Summary of the reproductive cycle: Days 1 to 28
Low estrogen and progesterone (1) reminds the hypothalamus to produce GRH (2) which stimulates the pituitary to release FSH (3). This stimulates the Graafian follicle to grow and make estrogen (4), which rises to a peak and advises the hypothalamus that it is ripe and ready for the next step. The hypothalamic surge of GRH (5) passes the message onto the pituitary and a surge of LH (6) releases the egg and causes formation of the corpus luteum. Progesterone and estrogen from the corpus luteum (7) lasts 14 days and then decreases (8), with formation of the corpus albicans, reminding the hypothalamus to start the whole cycle off once again.

respond. At this point the patient is postmenopausal. The above activity is shown in Figure 15.

The real difference after menopause therefore lies in the amount of hormone around. The most obvious feature is how much less estrogen is present in the postmenopausal woman compared to a fertile woman. This is shown in Figure 16.

What female sex hormones normally do for the body

What are estrogens and progesterone needed for anyway?

They have widespread effects on many parts of the body. Regard estrogen and progesterone, if you like, as builders of tissue. The more builders around, generally anyway in the body if not at the

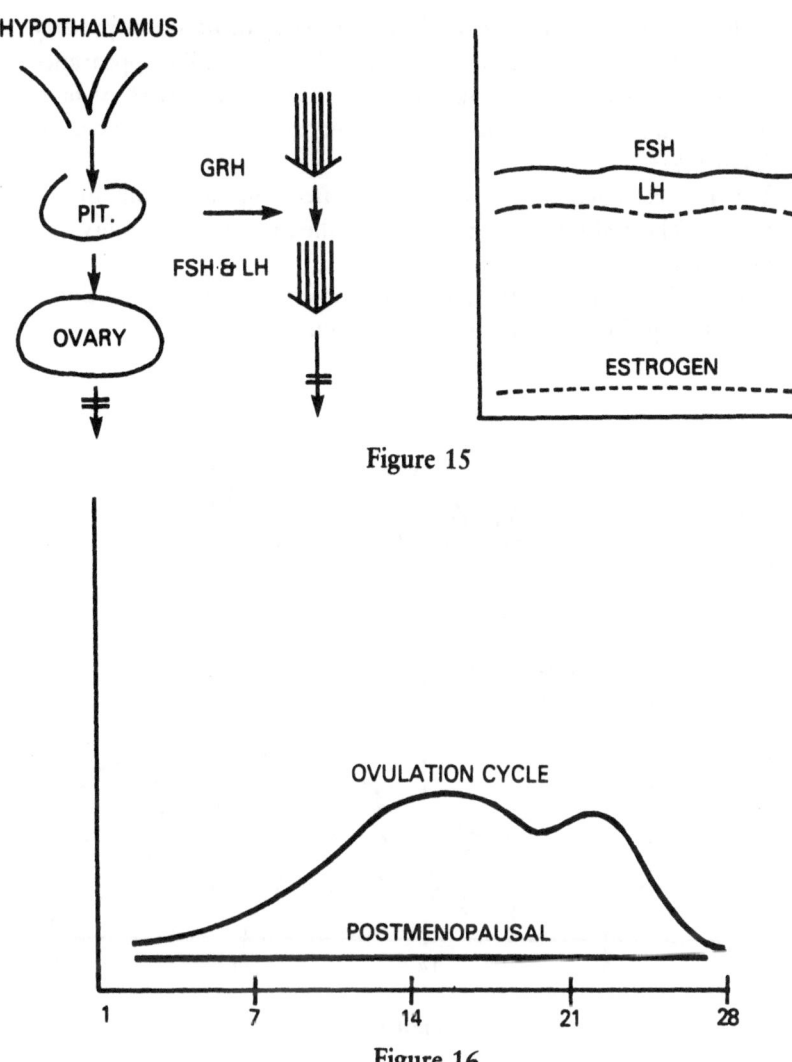

Figure 15

Figure 16

new schoolhouse, the more building that gets done. This is easier to grasp as an idea if we consider their effects on the actual parts of the body.

Direct effects on the sex organs
The names of the sex organs were described earlier in this book.

Vulva   With the onset of production of sex hormones at puberty the vulva undergoes a dramatic change. The flat slitlike appearance of the young child takes on the adult form with growth of hair, increase in size of the labia and slight increase in size of the clitoris (Figure 5).

Vagina   Estrogen has a stimulating effect on the lining of the vagina. The real effect is an increase in the thickness, pliability and potential sex function of the vagina.

Uterus   The lining of the uterus (endometrium) changes in thickness during the menstrual cycle as shown in Figure 17.

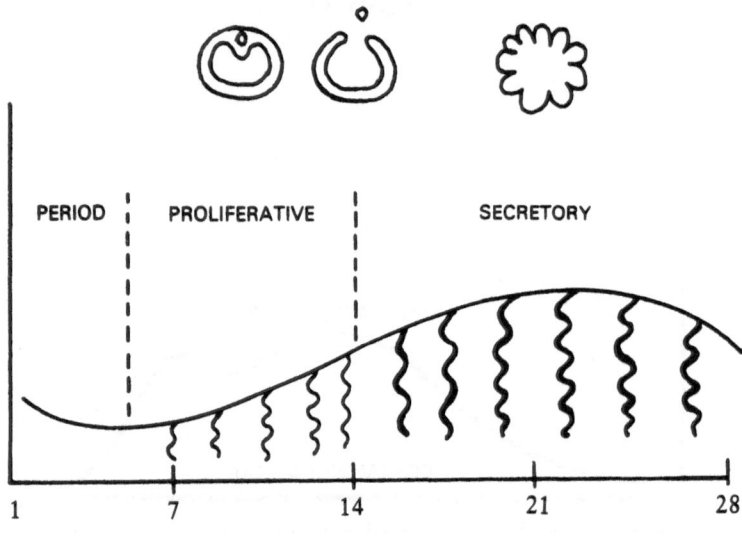

Figure 17

Estrogen should be regarded as a building contractor responsible for erecting the main shell of an apartment block. It thickens the lining of the uterus. Progesterone is the interior decorator who comes along and puts in all the finishing touches to make the place liveable. This effort at good housekeeping is aimed at creating a favourable environment for the fertilized egg.

These hormonal effects will occur irrespective of whether the hormones come from the ovary itself, or follow the taking of hormone tablets by mouth. Too much estrogen will cause too much thickening of the endometrium, and this can result in abnormal bleeding patterns. This lesson applies when we get to considering the use of estrogen treatment after menopause.

General bodily effects of estrogens
Normally estrogen and progesterone as builders and decorators, have many effects all over the body. After menopause with the loss of hormone, the effect on the tissues is lost as well. Sometimes the taking of hormones as medication may yield the same effects on the tissues as the natural hormones. All this will be explained in Chapter 6. At this point repetition would be superfluous. The following however is a list of the other parts of the body that respond to female hormones and that will eventually be considered:

1. Skin
2. Skeleton (bone)
3. Heart and blood vessels
4. Blood
5. Urinary tract – especially the bladder
6. Breast
7. Psychological behaviour.

Congratulations, you have just completed the most difficult chapter in the book. The rest should be a pleasure.

6 True effects of menopause and role of replacement hormones

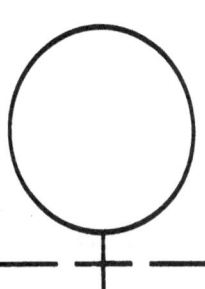

What to really expect after menopause and where hormone treatment can help

We now continue the saga of our two main characters, estrogen and progesterone.

Consider the scenario. Estrogen and progesterone have been in business as building contractors and interior decorators for over 35 years, from the woman's age of about 15 to 50. Unfortunately their financial support runs out and they disappear from the scene. The property they have previously cared for starts to decay. Our purpose will now be to examine the precise deterioration that occurs.

But we will do more than that. Estrogen and progesterone are hardy characters and lurk somewhere in the background. Their place of hiding is the drug store and the doctor's office. So we will examine too what possible good effects result from replacing these hormones as medical treatment.

Unfortunately, the story is complicated because estrogen has a sneaky side to it. When given as medical treatment it may produce unwanted effects. These will be considered in Chapter 7. Not surprisingly, the good and the bad news about estrogen has created the raging controversy as to whether it should be used or not. The pros and the cons and a balanced opinion will be presented in Chapter 12.

TRUE SYMPTOMS RELATED TO MENOPAUSE

Most modern medical textbooks still present long lists of symptoms due to menopause. It is often suggested that estrogen will alleviate them all. Little effort is made to look to the non-hormonal symptoms, that is, those that you will now recognize as the psycho-socio-cultural symptoms.

It should therefore come as no surprise to you to find that a modern list of early symptoms due to estrogen lack is very short.

True estrogen deficiency symptoms
Early

1. *Loss of periods* Loss of menstruation indicates menopause, but the periods should be absent for at least 8 to 12 months to clinch the diagnosis. If this occurs at a younger age, then other possible causes for loss of menstruation must be looked for before a diagnosis of menopause can be made. If in doubt, see your doctor.

2. *Hot flushes (flashes)* This is the classic symptom of climacteric and can occur several months before the actual menopause itself. The number and severity is extremely variable. They are described as a sudden feeling of heat in the face, neck and chest, and are brought on by excitement, nervousness, hot or spicy food, change in weather and almost any other stimulus. Following the flush, perspiration will develop and this may be followed by shivering or chill.

3. *Night sweats (perspiration)* Some people complain of waking during the night with bouts of perspiration and chill.

Later

Other symptoms can develop months to years after menopause and still be related to a shortage of estrogen. For example the vaginal lining becomes thin and easily subject to injury. Painful intercourse may result. Another example is that bone becomes thinner and can lead to backache or fracture. Details about these problems will be given when the individual parts of the body are discussed below.

Non-hormonal or psycho-socio-cultural symptoms

These are the symptoms that are caused by societal attitudes, the woman's environment and the strength or structure of her character. Thus many symptoms can be listed here like inability to sleep (insomnia), depression, headache, apprehension, irritability, mood changes, frigidity and so forth. This is an important group of symptoms of real concern to the woman, but they are not related directly to loss of hormones.

The treatment of menopausal symptoms

One important direction must be given to you. The doctor has to be certain that the symptoms are related to menopause and not the result of some disease that has arrived by coincidence at the same time. With this proviso in mind, treatment is simple. Symptoms due to lack of estrogen must be treated if possible with estrogen. The other symptoms need something else. Readers of this book could consider starting menopause support groups, or far better should take the advice offered in Chapter 13 in preference to non-hormonal medication including tranquilizers or to social and psychotherapy which ideally should be unnecessary.

The administration of estrogen is the responsibility of the physician, but some details for your own information are given in Chapters 8 and 9.

Some women cannot take estrogens, for the reasons given in Chapter 7, and the doctor may suggest non-hormonal medication. Such drugs include clonidine, sedatives and ergot alkaloids and are given as an alternate to relieve hot flushes. There is no reason why they should not be considered, but understand why they are given.

EFFECTS ON SKIN AND HAIR

After the menopause there is a gradual ageing of the skin and change in texture of the hair. Premature menopause brings this change on earlier.

Recently estrogen treatment has been shown to be of some value in reversing this effect and so it can be looked at as a possible advantage of such therapy.

BREAST CHANGES

Many women feel changes in their breasts during their normal monthly cycle. This is a result of the changing levels of the sex hormones. Loss of these hormones after menopause can result in smaller breasts. Fatter individuals will of course hardly notice the difference.

Estrogen treatment is not very good at restoring firmness to breasts. Moreover they can be risky if a lump is present. This means that you should always be sure to have your breasts checked at regular intervals, and in between checks should know how to do it yourself. Do not look to estrogen as a breast developer.

SEX ORGANS AFTER MENOPAUSE

The building effects of estrogen and progesterone were described in Chapter 5. Removal of these hormones sends everything into reverse. Thus the uterus gets smaller and the lining thinner. The lining of the vagina also gets thinner. The external genitalia may shrink and some pubic hair lost. The good news is that, except for the thinning of the vaginal skin, none of these changes are of any consequence in your life and will certainly not affect your sex life. Even the vagina is easily treated with local estrogen cream preferably, or else by mouth.

Sex hormones do have another pelvic function. They maintain the firm tone of the muscles of the pelvis. When the estrogen goes, this tone gets less and the uterus, bladder and vagina can drop to a varying degree. This condition is called *prolapse* and is illustrated in Figure 18. If the bladder descends it is called a *cystocele*. Prolapse of the rectum into the vagina is called a *rectocele*. Compare the normal anatomy in Figure 6 to the changes with prolapse in Figure 18.

Symptoms of prolapse are usually described as a 'feeling of something coming down' or else as a sense of heaviness. If the bladder is involved then coughing or laughing may cause a little urine to leak out despite the best of intentions to keep it in. This is called *stress incontinence*.

Fortunately there are highly successful treatments available.

1. Pelvic floor exercise helps very mild cases only but should be tried, even if just to strengthen the muscles before surgery. It simply involves contracting or tightening the pelvic muscles several times a day.
2. Extrogens can improve the muscle tone and are of value in mild cases.
3. Pessaries and rings are plastic devices inserted by the gynaecolo-

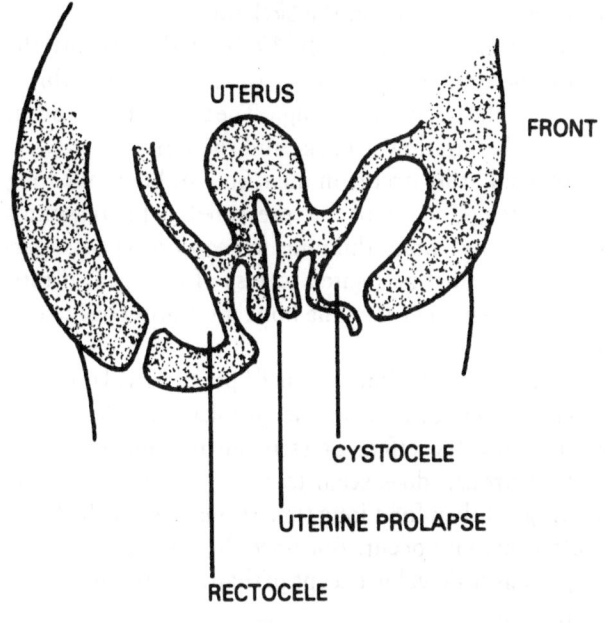

UTERUS

FRONT

CYSTOCELE

UTERINE PROLAPSE

RECTOCELE

Figure 18

gist to lift up the organs. They are used to delay surgery, or if the patient is too ill to undergo an operation.

4. Surgical repair is the best treatment. Because prolapse is not a disease, surgery must only be done if you have troublesome symptoms. Young women who want to further their family can have an operation where the uterus is saved. Otherwise the most effective results are obtained if the uterus is removed, an operation called *vaginal hysterectomy with repair*.

Remember that the most important function of the vagina is the enjoyment of an active and fulfilling sex life. Many women who feel that the vagina has become stretched and patulous, no longer offering the favourable sexual sensations to which they were accustomed, can look to vaginal repair operations. This is nothing to be embarassed about, and represents a vital aspect of your life.

FEMALE HORMONE AND THE SKELETON

If any single indication for long-term estrogen therapy exists, then it is in relation to its effects on the skeleton.

This story started in the early 1940s with a report that after menopause the bone started to get thinner and that this resulted frequently in the bone breaking. These fractures occur most frequently at the hip, lower back, and the wrist.

The problem hardly occurs in men. So it did not take long for an apparently 'logical' cure to be presented. The reasoning went something like this. Bone thinning (*osteoporosis*) developed after menopause so it must be related to loss of estrogen. If estrogen is given back to the patient then the bone must grow back, and be less liable to break.

The therapy enjoyed a long vogue of popularity. Unfortunately it did not cure osteoporosis. So the problem was looked at more closely, and now the effect of estrogen treatment is understood more fully. Estrogen does seem to prevent loss of bone. In other words, estrogen taken for a long time seems to slow the loss of bone that would otherwise occur. But once the bone is already reduced the estrogen has little value except perhaps to prevent the condition getting any worse.

Should all women be given estrogen because of these findings? The answer is not clear. The earlier menopause arrives, the greater the chance of a bone problem. So it is likely that a woman with premature menopause would be helped by estrogens.

Remember that there are other ways to assist bone growth. Exercise and good food are of prime importance, the former as a stimulation to growth and the latter to provide the blocks needed to build.

Much like sexual activity and the vagina, you are urged to use your body or lose it. Keep active, keep physically fit, keep moving.

HORMONES AND HEART DISEASE

The unpleasant reports of sudden death of a young person from a heart attack invariably involved men. It is not surprising therefore that many articles appeared in medical magazines suggesting that the woman before menopause had some factor that protected her against coronary accidents, and that this was absent in older women and men. It seemed that this factor must be estrogen. The story has not turned out to be that simple.

Early medical studies showed that young males have far more extensive disease affecting the blood vessels of their hearts than do females of the same age. Moreover, females undergoing premature or early menopause also showed these bad affects in the heart. This evidence does prove that the ovary does exert some protective effect on the blood vessels and the heart.

The facts given above can certainly be used as an argument in favour of saving ovaries at the time of surgery (see Chapter 10). Unfortunately it was also considered as more than sufficient evidence by some estrogen-forever believers to claim that such treatment after menopause prevented women from having heart attacks, and they carried on regardless.

No evidence came in to support their claims. Quite the opposite in point of fact. Estrogen, as used in the birth control pill, was reported as a possible cause for heart disease, especially in women over 40. Estrogen given to males who had survived a heart attack actually found their chances of having another attack *increased*. Then more precise measures of fats and other things in the blood that warn about heart disease showed that estrogens did not produce beneficial changes in the blood at all.

The result of all this is that estrogen is no longer considered a protective against blood vessel disease and heart attacks. Unfortunate, but true.

ESTROGEN AND MOOD

Finally, what about the effect of estrogen on the psyche or mind? Careful study has suggested that some women, usually the minority, have less energy after menopause and notice this as a decreased interest for work. There have even been claims for a reduction in intellectual performance at this time.

None of the above is proven. What is proven is that estrogen treatment after menopause makes many women feel better. There is a distinct elevation in mood. At one stage I did not believe this and prided myself that it was what physicians call T.L.C. (Tender Loving Care). Now I accept it as the mental tonic effect of estrogen.

7 Risks of hormone therapy

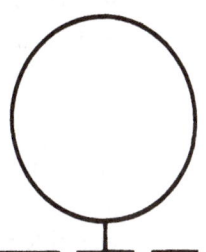

The sobering side of the situation

Remember the old joke that everything nice was either illegal, immoral or fattening? Well, estrogen replacement treatment also carries a bad news side.

The favourable side of the estrogen coin was exposed first. The result was the initial excessive and uncontrolled enthusiasm for its replacement. Virtually unabated, this continued until the end of 1975 when the use of estrogen was related to the risk of cancer of the uterus. Between 1964 and 1973 American women are said to have spent four times as much money buying estrogens as they had in the previous decade. The rate at which estrogen was selling through the early 1970s gave every indication that dramatic new sales records were going to be set.

The pendulum is now in danger of swinging to the opposite extreme. That is, there now exists the real possibility that women who need and should get estrogen will not be given it because of physician-fear or will not take it because of patient-alarm.

Part of the confusion can be blamed on the media. In the early days, particularly after the publication of *Feminine Forever* in 1965, the lay press was enthusiastic about the new estrogen therapy. Hundreds of superlatives were added to the numerous exaggerations that had already appeared in Wilson's book. Today these reports are quite to the contrary and women are warned off these hormones under almost all circumstances. The media of course do little more than reflect the confusion and disarray that exists within the medical profession itself.

The purpose of this chapter will be to give you an impartial analysis of the situation. The pendulum will be returned to mid-position. In the process you will be able to decide for yourself.

As a first step let me present you with an analogy. What would you say if a 3-year-old child was playing with acid and spilled some on a little friend, burning her in the process? You could hardly blame the child, nor could you blame the acid. You would of course try and find out how a child got hold of a dangerous substance and was able to play with it without supervision. Similarly, if a potent hormone like estrogen is used in uncontrolled fashion, you should look not only to the effects but also to how it was used and the controls that existed.

The problem about estrogen given for long periods of time, is that it was commenced with a fanfare of trumpets and a blast of promises before the basic necessary research had been completed. Looked at another way, virtually no medication exists in the world today that does not carry some risk in addition to the desired effect. But considerable animal and human research is undertaken first to find out what the risks and benefits are.

Estrogen, like acid, has potential dangers, but both have numerous practical values and uses. Provided due respect and control is observed there is no reason to withhold it from treatment. The following are the items that need to be listed in the debit column of the balance sheet you are drawing up concerning the risk to benefit ratio of estrogen therapy.

VAGINAL BLEEDING AFTER MENOPAUSE

Under normal circumstances, estrogen is the building constructor of the uterine lining. The more estrogen present, the thicker the endometrium. Withdrawal of the hormone results in the tissue losing its support and it is shed and comes away as menstrual flow.

Any form of bleeding from the vagina that occurs 6 months or longer after the menopause is called *postmenopausal bleeding*. This complication is unpleasant for the patient, and alerts the gynaecologist to the possible presence of something wrong.

After menopause, the normal decrease in amount of estrogen results in the uterine lining becoming very thin. But replacement of estrogen by any route can cause regrowth of the lining. The possibility of shedding and bleeding again becomes a reality.

The likelihood of postmenopausal bleeding occurring on

estrogen treatment depends on how much was taken and for how long. In all instances the possibility of this problem arising should be discussed with your doctor. In that way you can avoid being alarmed. Ask what he would do or suggest in the event of it happening. Many doctors will disregard the first event, but would invariably recommend a diagnostic curettage (D. and C. – also called womb scraping) for any subsequent events.

The condition of postmenopausal bleeding should never be ignored. It may be the first early warning of uterine cancer; it may not represent anything at all. Whether you are on estrogens or not, you should *always* report any episode of this type of bleeding to your doctor.

Postmenopausal bleeding is a nuisance; it does not represent a reason for not taking estrogen.

THE RISK OF BREAST OR UTERINE CANCER

Until the end of 1975 there was little reason to suspect estrogen as a cause of cancer of the breast or uterus. Some studies even suggested that fewer cancers might occur in patients on this treatment.

In December 1975 two articles appeared in the *New England Journal of Medicine* stating that the use of estrogen treatment seemed to be associated with an increased chance of developing a cancer in the uterus. Some months later another article in the same journal suggested an increased risk of breast cancer also to be possible, but as compared to uterine cancer the risk was not as great.

These articles stirred up a hornet's nest. Debate started among lay and medical circles and continues to this moment. The Food and Drug Administration in the United States felt the evidence strong enough to hold several enquiries. They ordered a warning to be printed on the package of every estrogen-containing product on the market.

But just how great is the risk?

The chance of *any* woman developing a cancer in the uterus after menopause is about 1 in every 1000. The risk of development of uterine cancer in women on estrogen therapy depends on how high the dose was and for how long it was taken. Also, if it was taken continuously instead of with monthly breaks, then the chance is increased. At the worst the risk with estrogen is increased to between 4 and 8 per 1000.

Perhaps these figures can be placed in better perspective by giving some comparable statistics. Estrogens increased the risk of uterine cancer 4 to 8 fold. Smoking 20 cigarettes a day increases the risk of death from lung cancer 17 fold. Driving a motor car in most major cities carries a risk of death by accident of about 35 per 100 000 per year.

The published articles came in for a lot of criticism ... not showing how much estrogen was taken ... little idea of how long ... cycled or continuous treatment ... whether there had been any progesterone added ... and so forth.

Most medical groups felt that no firm conclusions were warranted but nonetheless advised the exercise of caution. It does seem that estrogen in itself is probably not a direct cancer producer, but abused it can produce harmful effects. The active research that is under way will doubtless help resolve the dilemma in the not too distant future.

The following is the best advice that can be given to you until the answers become clear. A risk does exist. With modern usage this risk is likely to be small. Modern usage of hormone means the lowest dose, given in cycles (that is with regular breaks), and preferably with progesterone added to each cycle each month. You must be aware that the presence of certain conditions increases the risk to you as an individual. These are obesity, abnormal uterine bleeding, known disease of the breast including a family history of cancer, and even possibly cigarette smoking.

If you take estrogen therapy, you should do so with the clear understanding that this necessitates constant control by a physician whom you should see every 6 to 12 months. At these visits careful breast and pelvic examinations as well as cancer screening tests will be done.

Your doctor is as aware as you are of the dangers. Respect for estrogens and precautions in administration and follow-up will considerably reduce the risk. The evidence to date does not warrant their removal from medical usage.

THE RISK OF BLOOD CLOTS (THROMBOEMBOLISM)

If you think you have heard about all the possible dangers of estrogen, you had best sit yourself down in comfort and prepare to hear more.

Most women have been alerted to the dangers of the birth control pill (oral contraceptive). Did you know that this pill is simply a mixture of estrogen and progestin? Anyway, the most serious problem that can happen with the oral contraceptive is that the blood can clot in the veins of the leg. If a piece breaks off and travels to the lung it can block the circulation and cause sudden death. The chances are unusual in young patients and the incidence normally quoted is about 4 to 6 deaths per 100 000 women on the pill per year. Remember, again, that 35 per 100 000 people per year are likely to die on the roads.

Women over the age of 40 on the birth control pill take a much greater risk of getting this complication, and for this reason are advised against the pill. But estrogen after the menopause may also be at fault and so a little further comment is not out of place.

Certain situations, called *risk factors*, are associated with an increased chance of developing blood clots (thrombosis). These are obesity, high blood pressure, cigarette smoking, severe varicose veins and a previous history of thrombosis. Do you notice that obesity appears as a risk factor for the second time in a row? Take care and start a diet.

Certain of the brands of estrogen may be more at fault than others. Two types in particular are being looked into, namely ethinyl estradiol and methyl ethinyl estradiol. The most frequently prescribed estrogens are listed in Chapter 8.

The lessons for the woman considering estrogen treatment are fairly straightforward. The contra-indications to treatment must be respected, and the choice of drug is of importance.

LIVER PROBLEMS AND GALLSTONES

Some pregnant women complain of itchy skin. This occurs because of a certain effect of their high pregnancy levels of estrogen on the liver. This problem is most unusual with estrogen treatment but does show that this hormone has an effect on the liver. For this reason it should not be taken by anyone with liver disorders.

A most unexpected finding that has been reported is that women taking estrogens have a two and a half fold increase in chance of developing gallstones that require surgical treatment. The meaning of this observation is not clear.

One thought, however. Obesity is also associated with an increased incidence of gallstones. Medical textbooks describe the classical presentation of a patient with an inflamed gallbladder as being a 'female, fair, fat and forty'.

Have you started that diet yet?

MINOR SIDE-EFFECTS, EXPENSE AND INCONVENIENCE

This is the nuisance aspect of estrogen therapy. Of course, to one person a chore is a pleasure for another, and it is only possible here to provide a brief overlook.

Nausea is the most common side effect. It usually disappears after a few weeks. If necessary, contact your physician for an anti-nausea preparation (an anti-seasickness pill).

Water retention, or the holding back of fluid by the body, is recognized as a feeling of bloatedness, swelling of the legs, enlargement or sensitivity of the breasts, or as an increase in body weight. The problem usually settles by itself. The dose of estrogen may need to be reduced or even the preparation changed. Water losing tablets (diuretics) are *not* recommended medically as they can introduce their own set of problems.

Weight gain with estrogen means fluid retention. If there is weight gain and and no fluid retention then you are eating too much. Don't blame the poor old estrogen for everything.

Expense is a real factor. It is made up of three components. There are the physician visits, the laboratory follow-up tests and the actual cost of the drug itself. The burden of expense is clearly proportional to income and little can be gained by further discussion here. It is still too soon in terms of understanding long-term values of the hormone in disease prevention. The day may dawn where there is sufficient proof to justify large-scale estrogen use for prophylaxis of something like osteoporosis. In that event public health authorities will have to be made aware of the situation.

It is *inconvenient* to take a tablet almost every day. I can hardly remember to complete a course of antibiotics. But this is really a small effort for the return you expect, and will just have to become another daily habit.

WHEN ESTROGENS MUST NOT BE TAKEN

There are times when some treatments cannot be given to some people although others can take it with impunity. These are called *contra-indications*. In some instances this means *never*. In others it may mean *sometimes*. The never and the sometimes can only be resolved by an in-depth discussion with your physician. The list which follows is given by technical name without explanation. Hopefully, if you haven't heard of them then you haven't got them.

1. History of venous thrombosis
2. Present or previous cancer of the breast
3. Cancer of the uterus
4. Continuing liver disease or previous cholestatic jaundice
5. Chronic gallbladder disease
6. Abnormal hyperlipidaemias
7. Porphyria
8. Large uterine fibromyomata (fibroids)
9. Any estrogen dependent tumour
10. Dubin–Johnson's syndrome
11. Combination of obesity, varicose veins and cigarette smoking
12. Diabetes mellitus
13. Severe hypertension
14. Strong family history of breast or uterine cancer

Rules of complete therapy, 61

If a prescription is taken three times a day, this is reasonable ... make a complete ... but this is really a small effort for the reduced ... take it, it may have to become another daily habit.

WHAT TETRACYCLINES MUST NOT BE TAKEN

There are times when some treatments cannot be given ... some people although others cannot ... it works properly. These ... be under certain conditions. In some instances this never occurs ... it will be may even be very serious. The interest, and the sometimes you may be resolved by an in-depth discussion with your physician. The list which follows is given by technical name ... you're feeling. Hopefully, if you have a record of them that you haven't got them.

1. Allergy ... sensitivity
2. Present or recent ... ... kidneys
3. Cancer of the uterus
4. Continuing liver disease or recent or obstructive jaundice
5. Severe painful ... disease
6. Abnormal ... pigmentation
7. Porphyria
8. Enlarged ... or inflammatory disease
9. Any recent operation or other ...
10. Stroke, within the last year
11. Combination of estrogens which cause of certain medicine
12. Diabetes mellitus
13. ... hypertension
14. Pregnancy, within ... the ...

8 The frequently prescribed sex hormones

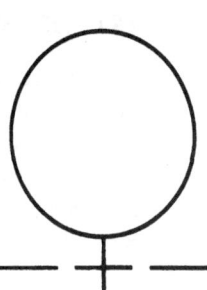

A bird's eye view of the hormones

It is clearly impossible to give you a full understanding of the use, effects and problems related to drug use in a short chapter. The intention is to simply provide a 'bird's eye view' of the more frequently prescribed products.

The only hormones to be considered will be the female sex hormones in the estrogen and progesterone category. The male hormone, testosterone, is not used very often in women anymore, fortunately, and will not be mentioned here again.

The words estrogen and progesterone are really the names for two groups of hormones and each can be sub-classified. Each of these sub-types have chemical names which are called in medical terms their *generic* names. These generic named drugs can be packaged or bottled separately or in mixtures, even with other drugs. The resultant commercial package lands up in the drug store with a different name called the *trade name*.

The generic names are internationally accepted; the trade names often differ country by country. Moreover, some drugs are available in some countries while others are not. The latter depends on local regulations and authorities, for example the Food and Drug Administration in the United States.

A way of checking out which type of hormone you are taking is to read the label on the bottle, or the descriptive leaflet inserted in the package. The trade name is generally printed in large fancy letters and the generic or chemical name in small letters below. This is also a way of looking for equivalent but cheaper-priced substitutes. The following names, then, are the generic or chemical names and not the trade names.

ESTROGENS

The estrogens that are available for clinical use are conveniently divided into three groups on the basis of their chemistry. The hormones listed below under Group A, that is the conjugated or natural estrogens, are usually considered preferable for use in treatment after the menopause. The substances listed under Groups B and C have specific and valued roles outside menopause therapy.

Estrogens available for clinical use

A Conjugated estrogens

These are often called the natural estrogens but may be derived from natural or synthetic sources. They include the following:

1. Conjugated equine estrogens
2. Esterified estrogens
3. Estradiol cypionate
4. Estradiol valerate
5. Estriol succinate or hemisuccinate
6. Piperazine estrone sulphate
7. Micronized 17β estradiol
8. Polyestradiol phosphate
9. Polyestriol phosphate

B Synthetic steroids — non-conjugated

These form the major components of the oral contraceptive.

1. Ethinyl estradiol
2. Methyl ethinyl estradiol (mestranol)
3. Quinestrol

C Synthetic non-steroids

1. Chlorotrianisene
2. Dienestrol
3. Diethyl stilbestrol

Combinations of estrogen with progesterone, tranquillizers or water-losing drugs are made. This is called polypharmacy, and is not generally in favour.

Tablets are preferable to injections or implants, the reasons being fully described in the next chapter

PROGESTERONES

Until the mid 1950s there were no preparations of progesterone available that were properly active when taken by mouth. The introduction of the orally active progesterone-like drugs (called *progestins*) had a historical impact, because this allowed the development of the birth control pill.

The addition of progesterone as a part of postmenopausal hormone treatment is now generally recommended because of the estrogen and cancer controversy. Progestin added to the estrogen therapy may result in a decreased chance of cancer developing, but this is yet to be proven. Keep an ear to the ground for further developments in this respect.

No major harmful effects additional to those for estrogen have been described in relation to the use of progesterone after the menopause. There is as yet no major reason for subdividing the different types of progestin that can be used at the menopause, so I will not burden you with the details.

WARNINGS

There are two final warnings about any form of drug use, and particularly potent hormones like estrogen and progesterone.

1. Do not medicate yourself. See a physician.
2. The full effects of virtually every drug in pregnancy are yet to be clarified. It has been emphasized before and is stated again – the diagnosis of menopause and the need for treatment must be determined before any drug therapy is considered. Missed periods can mean pregnancy.

9 Practicalities of the visit to the physician

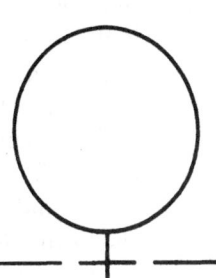

What to expect, what to do and what to ask

A medical check-up at regular intervals is an unfortunate but necessary fact of life, particularly after the age of 40. One advantage in your favour at this stage is that your new-found knowledge about menopause will help in the discussion you have with your physician about your health and your future. The purpose of this chapter is to brief you on what to expect and what to do when you see him.

Different doctors will do things in different sequence. They may recommend various tests. In general, the first step a doctor takes will be to get some idea of your overall state of health. He will ask many questions. So be prepared to provide a full and detailed medical history and to undergo a thorough physical examination. This will include a breast and pelvic examination. Certain tests will be performed including vaginal scrapings and cervical smears for hormone and cancer screening, and urine and blood tests under specific circumstances.

The physical examination is invariably the most dreaded part of the medical visit. Most women, however, are accustomed to a gynaecologic pelvic examination and realize that, although marginally uncomfortable, it should not be painful. If your doctor is hurting you, tell him. There is no reason for embarrassment. Pelvic examination is absolutely essential and cannot be avoided.

The usual technique of the pelvic examination is as follows. The external parts are inspected first for any problem, and then a warmed metal or plastic instrument called a speculum is gently passed into the vagina. This provides a direct view of the vagina itself, as well as the cervix. The opportunity is used to take the vaginal and cervical smears. Occasionally a specimen for bacterial culture will be taken as well.

The speculum is withdrawn and the bimanual pelvic examination follows. The doctor inserts two fingers of his gloved hand into the vagina and his other hand is placed on the lower aspect of the abdomen. He then proceeds to feel the cervix, uterus and ovarian areas between his hands. This is illustrated in Figure 19. In this way

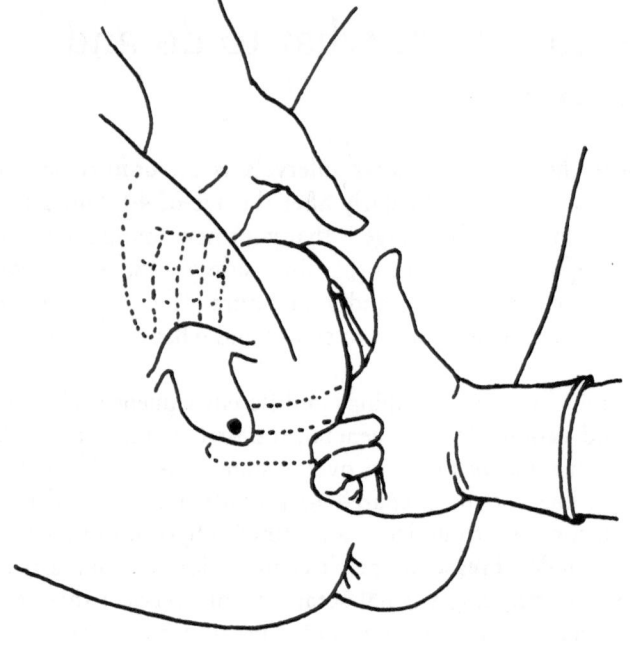

Figure 19

it is possible to detect enlargements of organs, tumours or cysts of the ovary, areas of tenderness and so forth. The whole pelvic examination rarely takes more than a few minutes.

While you dress, the doctor writes his medical notes, as they comprise an extremely important aspect of the consultation and will be referred to at every subsequent visit. When you re-join him he will expect you to raise questions and discuss any proposed treatment. Do not be afraid or hesitant to voice personal problems as they provide the doctor with further insight into your overall case and his broad experience will often result in concrete suggestions being made.

It is in vogue in some circles to regard the gynaecologist as being the extreme male chauvinist. This is unfair, and direct questioning of most women confirm their gynaecologists, both male and female, to be concerned people with the direct interests of their patients at heart. An honest, on-going patient–gynaecologist relationship proves for many women to be a deeply valued life experience.

If you request hormone treatment, the physician will be influenced by the following points:

1. Whether you have passed the menopause
2. A normal breast and pelvic examination
3. No contra-indications to hormone therapy
4. The degree of estrogen deficiency, usually measured by the severity of symptoms. A hormonal smear test is also useful.
5. The desires and motivation expressed by yourself. This is your moment to put questions and discuss doubts.
6. Alternative treatments other than hormones.

If you decide to take hormones and there is no reason against this, then two practical considerations will occupy the doctor's attention: the selection of drug or drugs (see Chapter 8) and the route by which the hormones are to be taken. Medication by mouth is generally to be preferred because:

1. It is painless.
2. It is safer. Treatment can be stopped abruptly in the event of the onset of side-effects.
3. It is cheaper. Injections and implants mean extra visits to the doctor.
4. The dosage can be adjusted on a day to day basis.
5. It is more physiological. An on-off-on regime (cyclical) is the method of choice and the oral route is the only practical one in this instance.

The doctor will advise on when to take the hormone tablets. A frequent practical recommendation is for the estrogen tablets to be taken from the first to the 25th day of each month, and no tablets at all for the rest of the month. If progestin tablets are also to be taken, these will usually be given as an additional tablet for the final 7 days of each estrogen course.

If you have trouble remembering when to take tablets, then mark the whole course out on a calender and check off each day you complete.

Regular check-ups are essential for any patient on treatment. These should be half-yearly or yearly, and will entail a similar pattern to the first visit. Your response to the hormones and the development of any side-effects will be considered. You should use this opportunity to discuss any problems and clarify any queries that you may have.

The following checklist, modified from '*Oestrogen Therapy*' by Doctor Pieter van Keep of the International Health Foundation and Professor Arey Haspels of the University of Utrecht, is reproduced with permission of *Excerpta Medica*. These are the usual steps taken at the medical examination and follow-up.

List of important factors in the first examination and check-ups

History
Presenting symptoms or complaints

Family history
Heart disease
Cancer of the breast, uterus or cervix
Diabetes

Personal history
Menopausal age/menstrual pattern
Particulars of pregnancies
Gynaecological operations
Vaginal bleeding
Breasts
Heart disease
Thromboembolic processes
Liver disease
Diabetes
Allergy and contra-indications to drugs
Family relationships and personal problems

Current disorders
Menopausal:
  Hot flushes
  Bouts of perspiration
  Palpitations
Psycho-socio-cultural:
  Nervousness, irritability, headache,
  insomnia, depression, etc.
Other factors:
  Stress incontinence or prolapse
  Vaginal irritation
  Aches in bone or joints
Sexual relations:
  Frequency
  Satisfaction
  Pain
  Change in interest or desire

General physical examination — note especially
Blood pressure*
Height and weight*
Breasts (mammography if necessary)***
Condition of skin, scalp hair, face, genitalia*

*Pelvic examination**

Laboratory examination
Urine for sugar and protein*
Blood for anaemia**
Cancer screening**
Hormone index on vaginal smear**

*should be repeated at every check-up examination
**should be repeated once yearly
***family history, age, physical examination etc. will determine
frequency of re-mammography

10 Surgery as a cause early menopause

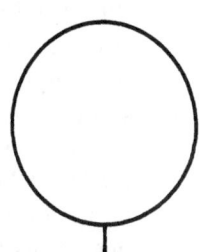

The fate of the ovaries at hysterectomy – leave them or remove them

Can you be postmenopausal and not know it? You most certainly can.

This chapter concerns one group of women who often tend to be forgotten. These women have been precipitated into early or premature onset of menopause and climacteric by removal of their ovaries during surgery, an operation called bilateral oophorectomy or ovariectomy. This procedure is usually performed at the time of removal of the uterus at surgery (hysterectomy). Many gynaecological surgeons consider this no more than a routine part of the operation.

Removal of the ovaries amounts in fact to castration. Because of the suddeness of the procedure the postmenopausal problems that follow are usually more severe than with spontaneous menopause. The author firmly believes, although both a male and a gynaecologist, that if more females had been gynaecologists, less patients would have undergone premature castration. It is therefore pertinent and timely to take a long, lean look at this procedure for the reasons behind it and for situations where it should or should not be done. Once again, the history is of interest.

In 1685 Justice Theodorus Schorkopff suggested that ovarian lumps (cysts) should be removed 'provided the operation were not too cruel or hazardous'. He did not perform the operation however. The year 1809 marked a milestone in abdominal surgery when Ephraim McDowell, after 14 years of medical practice in the frontier town of Danville, Kentucky, successfully performed the first surgical removal of an ovarian cyst. He realised the procedure was experimental. For many years the medical profession in general failed to give approval. But the word got around. Charles Clay (1801–1893), called the 'father of ovariotomy' in Britain because he performed the first operation in 1842, did so many of these operations that he used to reckon his performances by the ton, thinking nothing of referring to 2000 pounds by weight removal of ovarian tumours per month.

Robert Battey (1828–1895) in 1872 was the first to remove both ovaries for conditions like painful periods (dysmenorrhea) and neuroses. He attempted to justify the operation of removal of normal ovaries by stating: 'The removal of both ovaries puts an end to ovulation entirely and this determines the menopause or change of life; whereby I have hoped, through the intervention of the great nervous revolution which ordinarily accompanies the climacteric, to uproot and remove serious sexual disorders and re-establish the general health'. In mitigation he did add: 'I believe these organs should alone be sacrificed for grave causes, and then only as a dernier resort, when the hitherto recognised resources of our art have been expended in vain'.

Despite the passing of years heated controversy still exists among doctors as to the justification for the procedure.

The usual reasons given for removal of ovaries at the same time as hysterectomy are as follows:
1. To prevent the later development of cancer in the ovaries if they are left behind.
2. A theory that ovaries left behind after hysterectomy do not work properly.
3. The possible need for surgery at a later date to remove ovarian cysts.

The ovaries are frequently saved in order to:
1. Prevent the symptoms which normally follow their removal.
2. Prevent possible changes in other body organs because of loss of ovarian hormones, for example breasts, skin and vagina.
3. Prevent thinning of bone (osteoporosis).

4. Prevent earlier onset of heart attacks (coronary thrombosis).
5. The psychological reasons.

The effects on the body following early removal of normal ovaries were discussed in Chapter 6. As far as we know, normal ovaries retained at the time of surgery do far more for the female than any form of hormone replacement therapy.

The most important reason given for removing ovaries is the possible risk of cancer developing in the ovaries if they are left behind. You say that is a pretty good reason? I agree. Unfortunately the medical literature cannot tell us how frequently this is liable to happen. The most reliable statistics point to this risk being somewhere between 1 in 1000 to about 1 in 3000 hysterectomies. This will mean that some 999 to 2999 women would have to be castrated in order to prevent one case of ovarian cancer. Admittedly no one wants to be the statistic. On the other hand the evidence that will be mentioned later as to the protective effect of the ovary in the development of serious problems like heart disease and bone fractures must be taken into account.

The argument sometimes given that ovaries left behind after hysterectomy do not work is just not true. Except for the most unusual circumstances they will normally continue to function until the originally expected time of menopause.

WHEN SHOULD OVARIES BE REMOVED?

There are times when the ovaries have to be removed despite the best intentions. These are as follows:

1. If the woman is passed menopause. The ovaries have clearly ceased to function, and there is little to justify leaving them behind. This applies irrespective of age.
2. If she is premenopausal but over the age of 50. Menopause is going to occur fairly soon, and the ovary has little future.
3. If the surgeon considers the ovaries to appear abnormal or diseased at the time of surgery. This means giving open consent to the doctor – but if you have discussed the possibility with him before surgery he will realise the value you place on your ovaries.
4. If the surgery is being performed for pelvic cancer, for example uterine cancer. In this instance it is likely that the ovaries would

have been subjected to x-irradiation before surgery, or will be so managed after surgery, and this would destroy the ovaries anyway.
5. The wishes of the patient. If a patient wants her ovaries removed then that is her prerogative. However she should be aware of the consequences.
6. If it is surgically impossible to save the ovaries. This possibility will arise in some patients with a long history of pelvic infection.

It is very clear that every woman about to undergo abdominal surgery should discuss the fate of her ovaries with the doctor. Remember that it is your own body and future under discussion, and the decision taken holds long-term implications for yourself. You have the right to withhold consent for any procedure additional to the intended one, and should exercise this right if no substantial reason can be presented to you for its being undertaken.

In conclusion, the surgeon and the patient should respect the ovary for the functioning endocrine gland that it is and only agree to its removal once all the for and against arguments have been considered. The author is a strong conservative in this respect.

SOMETHING ABOUT HYSTERECTOMY ITSELF

The procedure of hysterectomy or removal of the uterus can be performed without removing the ovaries.

The uterus has two roles, acting as a container for pregnancy and a source of the monthly menstrual bleeding. Hysterectomy is therefore followed by loss of fertility and loss of periods. These two events aside, uterine removal should have little affect in the long term.

There is one proviso to the above. Prior to surgery a woman should discuss all doubts she may have with her physician. The unprepared patient shows an increased chance of losing interest in sex. The emotionally prepared patient develops quite the opposite attitude. The following poem aptly reflects this:

HALLELUJAH TO HYSTERECTOMY
or
(Let's stop talking about sex and do something about it)

Speak to me not of birds and bees
Of the passion of flowers keep mum
About the amorous habits
Of snakes and rabbits
I prefer from now on to stay dumb.

In my day I have functioned with no little success
As a human producer ad nauseam
But my last trump is played
I was recently spayed
Of the vital organs which causeam.

In future, my thoughts will be mostly concerned with
Things — spiritual, social, intellectual
Three cheers. Jubilation.
I'm past pollination
With a brand new outlook sexual.

I can plan strenuous trips any time of the month
I can tweak my husband at random
To that Doc with a knife
Who has so changed my life,
A magnum of brandy, I'll hand 'm.

And all I can say to my gal friends is this . . .
Hysterectomy's the one bed of roses
For gals over forty
Who, tho' still feelin' sporty
Loathe the contraptions of Bessie Moses.

(By a patient of a doctor-friend of the Editor
of Obstetrical and Gynecological Survey.
Reprinted with the permission of the Editor
and the Publishers, The Williams and Wilkins Co.)

11 Sexual activity after the menopause

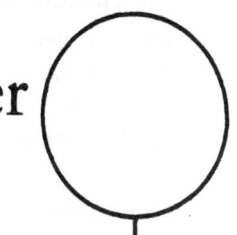

Do you or don't you and are there any limitations or risks?

A major part of the fun after menopause is that you can indulge in sexual intercourse to your heart and body's content without there being any fear of pregnancy. Yet, unfortunately, so few make the most of this wonderful opportunity. Masters and Johnson are often quoted as saying 'use it or lose it'. But how many heed this advice?

If one were to listen to the popular fallacies about sexual performance and enjoyment in older age, the future would be distressing to think of. 'Males start their decline after the age of 18 and females after 30'. Let whoever said that speak for herself/himself. I do not believe that and neither should you. Sexual activity is for all, and is most definitely not the prerogative of the young. Moreover, the adage that 'experience counts' is true for everything, sexual ability and enjoyment included.

The sexual myths surrounding ageing are superbly dealt with by Margaret Kuhn in a multi-authored book called *Sex and the Life Cycle* (Grune and Stratton, New York, 1976) and to which readers looking for an in-depth discussion are referred. She lists five sexual myths, which are briefly as follows:

1. Sex does not really matter in old age and the later years of life are sexless anyway.
2. For old people to be interested in sex is abnormal.
3. Remarriage after the death of the husband should be discouraged.
4. It is ridiculous for old women to be sexually involved with

younger men although it is fine for an old man to seek a younger sex partner.

5. The sexes should be separated in institutions to avoid problems for the staff or criticism by families and the community.

Five fallacies out of a fund of dozens that could be gleaned from the literature. All perpetuated, all believed by many and all totally wrong on all counts.

The blame for the negative image of sex after middle age rests squarely on the shoulders of societal attitudes and the media. The clichés of the 'gay young blade' versus the 'dirty old man' and of the 'jet-set young model' versus the 'silly old woman' must be erased from the records and a new set of standards based on human rights irrespective of sex and age needs development. Let us see TV commercials for sexy senior citizens and hear of positive experiences of 80-year-olds.

It is untrue that sex is not needed in old age, and that interest in sex is abnormal for old people. Sexual response is a fundamental part of human physiology. People are aware of their genitalia, their own needs, general sexual interest, arousal and behaviour every day, just as they have an appetite to eat.

Organic illness or emotional shock can blunt the sexual response in exactly the same way as it would affect the appetitite. But once the illness or shock is over the normal healthy sex needs will resurface, provided they are not constantly repressed by embarrassment for what people will think and other unreal societal attitudes.

By the same token, remarriage after the loss of a spouse should be encouraged. To live alone is extremely difficult for most people, and this is even more so for someone accustomed to human warmth and company. Adult children that oppose re-marriage generally do so on selfish grounds, and cannot have their parents welfare at heart. Moreover, companionship and marriage are not irreparably bound or mutually exclusive. It is acceptable socially to live together, and marital status is your own business anyway.

The onus is on you the individual to keep yourself open to human contact and not to be adversely influenced by certain societal norms no longer pertinent to the modern era.

The human body does show physiological or functional changes in sexual response in relation to age. As the woman gets older, vaginal lubrication may be reduced or slower, and greater stimulation will be required. This is not an abnormality, and pleasurable precoital foreplay is the obvious remedy. The actual orgasmic phase may be shorter, but there is no impairment in the capacity to have orgasm or even multiple orgasms.

The vulval and vaginal skin may cause discomfort because of an increased liability to injury. But this aspect, you' will no doubt recall, responds excellently to local estrogen therapy. So from a physical standpoint no impediment really exists to full sexual activity.

One detail bears repetition. Stretch of the vagina and pelvic floor after menopause is a real possibility and can reduce genital contact and satisfactory stimulation. This problem was discussed in Chapter 6. If vaginal stretch negatively affects sexual response a carefully planned and performed vaginal repair operation should remedy the situation. Do not be embarrassed to see a gynaecologist about this condition.

Actual problems about sexual performance (sexual dysfunction) can occur at any age. The present book makes no pretense at being a manual on sexual dysfunction and full details will not be dealt with. Ethical sex therapists and gynaecologists or psychiatrists specializing in sexual dysfunction now exist in most centres, and age is not a precluding factor in seeking their services. A negative attitude that 'it's too late' or 'doesn't matter anyway' is completely out of order. If your motorcar is malfunctioning, irrespective of it's age, you would take it in for repair. At least treat yourself with the same respect.

Do remember that contraception is necessary until the periods have disappeared for at least six months. Contraceptive advice at this time of life is best obtained from a physician. It is probably wiser to avoid the oral contraceptive after the age of 40. So this practically speaking leaves the choice between:

1. Intra-uterine devices. This is a good method, provided that there is no irregular bleeding, in which instance medical advice and it's removal becomes unavoidable.
2. Vaginal diaphragm and contraceptive foam/gel/creams. This is the most frequently used method at this time of life and certainly the best for your health.

82

3. Condoms. These are second best to the diaphragm for both the male and the female, as there is reduced sensation.

4. The other methods are really impractical.

In conclusion, please believe me, sexual activity is a basic human requirement. It is normal from youth until death. It is necessary for your physical and mental health. Human contact is always needed. Sexual activity provides that link and is the crutch against loneliness. If you have never had a positive attitude to sex, then start to foster one now or seek help. This is not a call for feckless promiscuity. It is a call for an honest and rewarding one-to-one relationship which will provide mutual comfort and support, benefit you health-wise, sustain you emotionally and save you from disintegrating alone.

12 An overall perspective

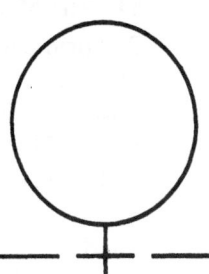

Do menopause and ageing mean the same thing? What aspects are preventable and what do I do?

Like astronauts before 'blast-off', you have now been fully briefed. You have read the facts about menopause, and the fallacies. We can now look to the final two steps. Step one, in this chapter, is to summarize and put in perspective the important components already presented. Step two, the subject of the next and final chapter, is the final advice about what to do. Hopefully you will transform that into a big stride into the future. But first the perspective.

During the reproductive age or time of fertility, usually between 15 and 50 years of age, the ovary produces eggs and hormones, notably estrogen and progesterone. The ovary eventually runs out of eggs and the production of estrogen and progesterone is consequently decreased. The final menstrual period signifying the end of this age of fertility is called the menopause, and the whole time around this event, before and after, is called the climacteric.

The individual proceeding through this event may develop symptoms or complaints and this is then referred to as the climacteric (postmenopausal) syndrome.

Symptoms or complaints of the climacteric syndrome are the result of inter-action between any or all of four possible components:

1. Hormonal alterations. These are specifically hot flushes as an early feature, or subsequent long-term changes in body organs that are deprived of estrogen and progesterone.

2. Socio-cultural factors directly influence the environment in which the woman finds herself at this time, and determine her own positive and negative responses to menopause and its supposed image. That is, positive factors favour less menopausal problems and *vice versa*.

3. Psychological factors reflect the actual structure of the woman's mind. Once again positive attitudes can produce significant benefits, whereas a negative personality is likely to result in a major psycho-somatic (mind over body) component to symptom formation.

4. The general ageing process continues unabated from fertilization until death. Concurrent illness or pathology can occur at any time, sometimes inevitable and sometimes the consequence of abuse of the body, for example cigarette smoking or obesity. The ageing process, outside of illness, is slow and plays little role in symptom production at or around the menopause. You really are as old as you feel.

The majority of women pass menopause with little obvious problem. Some 10 to 15 per cent however develop sufficient symptoms to seek medical care. Those women who develop problems severe enough to have the climacteric syndrome need a full medical check-up of their symptoms to decide precisely which follow hormone loss, and which are due to the other possible factors enumerated above.

The treatment of the symptoms depends entirely on the cause. Features due to lack of hormone, like hot flushes, justify estrogen treatment. In this instance the estrogen should be given in the lowest effective dose for the shortest duration of time needed to solve the problem. The other symptoms need to be treated according to the actual reason they developed in the first place.

The role of Menopause Clinics in larger medical institutions or Menopause Support Groups established by interested and concerned women themselves, was emphasized right at the beginning of the book. These offer support and services directly to the individual who is most in need. It is to be hoped that they will undertake another important task as well, and that is to change unacceptable societal attitudes, irrespective of their level of existence.

For a decade, from about 1965 to 1975, the climacteric in its entirety was considered by some to result from estrogen lack alone. A *Forever Feminine* approach with long-term estrogen therapy was advocated by some physicians on the one hand, and demanded by some women and the media on the other.

Abuse of the potent therapeutic hormones, estrogen especially, resulted in reports about harmful effects. For example, the possible relationship between estrogen and uterine cancer. At present the pendulum of popular opinion and the media is swinging in the opposite direction and away from this form of treatment. Potential users are calling for answers.

One of the purposes of this book has been an attempt to provide the degree of insight necessary to consider the possible advantages and disadvantages without prejudice or emotion.

Fortunately, ever since the mid-1960s, many medical researchers from all corners of the globe have been giving increased attention to the menopause, sex hormones and related problems. Initially the efforts were isolated, but gradually the answers to problems have been forthcoming. Not all the questions have been solved, and surprises are still inevitable. Nonetheless it is possible to draw up a balance sheet of probable benefits and possible risks and present you with the so-called risk to benefit ratio.

The possible BENEFITS of hormone replacement include
1. Relief of specific hormone-related symptoms.
2. Improvement in skin quality and hair texture.
3. Restoration of the vaginal epithelium and the base of the bladder to a healthy pre-menopausal state.
4. Prevention of deterioration of the skeleton by the thinning of bone, which could lead to fractures if left untreated.
5. A mental tonic effect, suggesting that patients on these hormones feel mentally more alert, and are less likely to develop mental impairment with age.

The possible RISKS of hormone treatment include
1. An increased likelihood of uterine bleeding after menopause.
2. The increased chance of developing breast or uterine cancer.
3. The chance of developing blood clots.
4. Several minor side effects including nausea, fluid retention and so forth.

5. The expense related to medical check-ups, special tests and purchase of the hormones.

6. The inconvenience of having to undergo more frequent check-ups than would usually be necessary, and of taking tablets almost every day.

In mitigation of the potential dangers, it does seem as if those reported thus far were the result of previous overuse or even misuse of estrogen. The future use of cyclical treatment in the lowest effective dose with added progesterone may yet prove to be remarkably safe. Only time and well planned and controlled studies will prove this point. With the facts you have already been given, and a balanced assessment of facts you gather in the future, you may yet be able to write a postscript to this chapter yourself.

Contraindications do exist to the use of estrogen and progesterone. Every patient contemplating this treatment must be aware of the need for physician control, and regular follow-up examinations and tests.

The decision as to whether or not you will commence such therapy is finally yours alone to make. Present indications are that the potential benefits outweigh the possible risks, but the precautions outlined in this book must be fully observed. There are no shortcuts and these are not rules to be broken.

Above all, one fact must be repeated and emphasized again and again. The climacteric has more to it than just a hormone component. Numerous other factors operate in the overall picture, so don't look at it in a narrow context only.

Menopause may be a milestone along the road of passing years, but it is also a reminder to use every remaining year, month and day wisely and without waste. Enjoyment of the next exciting leg of life's journey is the message of the final chapter.

13 Life after menopause

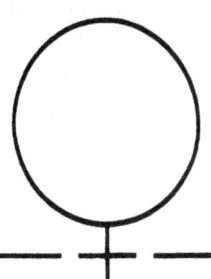

Now is the time to get up and go

The book is coming to an end. For many of you I sincerely hope and trust that this chapter will prove to be the beginning of something new, promising, exciting and rewarding.

Over 10 years involvement with women at the perimenopause proved for me to be more than a period of medical service. It became increasingly apparent that there was no average woman and no average response to menopause. There was one striking phenomenon that did become all too obvious. Motivation, drive, determination, grit or whatever you will call it, was directly related to the quality of life women were enjoying. I discussed attitudes with them, and herein lies the secret and the solution. A positive attitude was something that could be cultivated and developed.

The lesson was clear. Aggressive development of a positive frame of mind could lead directly to improvement in quality of life and the enjoyment of it. This is the GET UP AND GO philosophy, and the purpose of the following paragraphs is both to explain it and to inspire you towards determined and positive action.

The GET UP AND GO philosophy has three crucial components: the *principles* involved; the *tools* at your disposal; the *actions* to be taken.

THE PRINCIPLES INVOLVED

1. You are important, you are wanted and you are needed

'Me needed? Me wanted? Me important? Nonsense.' Nonsense indeed. But on your own part by your own devaluation of yourself. Self-pity will get you nowhere. The man in your life has problems in his life too and needs a positive influence. Negative attitudes will only pull you both down. He does need you and want you. And if no partner exists, a recognition of your own worth will help you find one. Your children too need you as much as ever, even if it is only to help bolster their own egos. If you are alone, you are important to yourself, and need yourself above all.

So do not under-estimate your worth – it is considerable.

2. You have more experience

Of course you are a little older, but that makes you a little wiser, and a lot more experienced. Draw on that experience.

Think back to the frustrations suffered by the teenager, and how much more effectively you would have dealt with problems then, if you only had the experience you have now. You would probably have been a menace.

3. You owe something to yourself

To most women, the years between 25 and 45 are an endless dedication and devotion of life, effort and spirit to husband and children. All too often the family takes as a right what is really an enormous privilege. By the age of menopause the children are grown and independent; husband is at the peak of his career or even beginning to ease off. This is now the time to take stock and reassess what is happening in your own life. One fact becomes immediately obvious to all but the naive. You have given of yourself to all but yourself.

Well, the time has come for you to put your foot down. So far and no further. You owe yourself a little something. This is not selfishness. It is consideration of self. The attitude is correct and the sooner you realize this, the sooner you can get on with improving the quality of the rest of your life.

4. You are as old as you allow yourself to feel

Many of the clichés of language are true – but none more true than that stating you are as old as you feel. Despite health problems, some chronically ill people impress everyone with their joyful exuberence. Many elderly people, healthy or otherwise, are enormous fun to be with. Others think, talk and feel 'old'. It is apparent that health is not the all-important factor, but that attitude is, and being a state of mind, it can be influenced. It is therefore more factual to say that 'you are as old as you allow yourself to feel'.

5. Time flies – each passing day is one less left to live

The fleeting passage of time can be viewed negatively as a depressing thought. It must be viewed from another perspective. Make the most of your time. Use it effectively and do not waste it.

6. If you have the money, then spend it on yourself

Many older parents take the defensive if advised to spend time and particularly money on themselves. 'There will be nothing left to leave for the children'. Utter nonsense. The children have been reared to independence. Any legacy other than that is a bonus. For the moment you must certainly look to your own retirement with security. But any cream left on top is for you yourself.

7. Ignore societal attitudes that are outdated

You should by now be fully aware that virtually all negative attitudes to menopause within a society are fallacies. Therefore ignore them. More than that, discredit them by your very actions. Show them to be the untruths that they are. Use your influence within the community to change the media and urge them towards a positive image of older people.

8. Enjoyment of life is not a sin

Which ever way you look at it, you are not harming anyone by having fun.

THE TOOLS AT YOUR DISPOSAL

1. Yourself

In essence you are the worker and the tool and the object of their efforts. This is a fact, and will become more obvious as we proceed.

2. Total body care

The care you devote to yourself is in direct proportion to your likelihood of success. The judicious use of cosmetics, with or without the beauty parlour, is important. Remember your hair.

These and other factors create the appearance, the model, the self-image so necessary to a high rating by yourself of yourself.

Let us enumerate these aspects for completeness:

1. General body hygiene
2. Oral and dental hygiene – your mouth and teeth
3. Care of the hair
4. Care of the skin – judicious use of cosmetics
5. Care of the nails
6. Regular medical check-ups.

3. Correct diet

A full, nutritious, well-balanced diet is important, and common sense tells what is good and what is bad. Avoid junk foods. If you are overweight, then diet. Obesity is due to overeating, and in itself carries a multiplicity of disadvantages, both to appearance and comfort as well as to health and longevity.

A common-sense weight reducing diet is presented in Appendix I, and is given with full acknowledgement to the Department of Dietetics at the Groote Schuur Hospital in Cape Town. This diet is well-balanced, and duly observed will produce consistent weight loss. If you cheat, only you are the victim.

4. Hormone treatment

This aspect has been amply dealt with. Decide for yourself whether you want them, and indeed whether you need them. But see them within the overall context of the present discussion.

5. Clothes that suit you

Correct dress is of extreme importance. Dress the role you decide to play but do not miscast yourself. Fashion is an individual preference. Look at your clothes impartially, and choose what is appropriate. If you have the figure for blue jeans and you prefer them, then wear them; but avoid extremes. The European woman tends to favour chic high-fashion and plays the sophisticated role. Look to what best suits you.

6. The physician

Medical advice and care is another tool to be used. Do not expect miracles; but do not ignore the modern medical treatments available nor the sound advice that a good on-going relationship with an interested physician can produce. Modern litigation-prone attitudes, particularly in the United States, have tended to diminish the image of the physician and the role he can play. This is a pity. I suggest you use your physician's counsel wisely.

7. Physical fitness

You need to be physically fit in order to be strong enough to take effective action. The dictum that a healthy mind in a healthy body applies. First see your physician for a medical check-up, advising of your intentions, and then start an appropriate method of exercise leading to physical fitness. There are several possibilities, examples being:

1. Health studios – advisable if you need constant encouragement and guidance.

2. Home physical fitness plans. These take self determination; boredom is the most frequent reason for stopping. The Royal Canadian Air Force exercise programme (Physical Fitness – XBX 12-minute a day plan for women. R.C.A.F., Penguin Books) is the plan I personally favour most. Whatever plan you choose, keep at it.

3. Sport. Tennis, yoga, golf, and similar sports are excellent exercise and the social contact is an added bonus. They are not usually sufficient for full physical fitness and should be additional to a specific exercise programme.

4. Swimming is a special sport and a few hundred metres up and down the swimming pool is a good way to fitness.

5. Sexual intercourse, scientifically speaking, is also a form of exercise, but a physical fitness exercise programme is still recommended, even if only to improve your sexual stamina. It is not true that sex is a common cause for death in older people, and even recent victims of heart disease are being encouraged to return early to a normal sex life.

8. Menopause clinics or menopause support groups

If you need that extra little bit of encouragement, then get it through a Menopause Clinic or a Menopause Support Group. If no such facility exists in your area, why not be the initial motivator to get one started? You will be doing yourself and others a big favour.

TAKE IMMEDIATE POSITIVE ACTION

1. Take an impartial look at yourself

Find a full-length mirror. Stand in front of it and take an impartial look at yourself. Be critical, but be fair and honest.

Do you like what you see?

If you were sitting at a sidewalk cafe in Paris and you saw this person go by, what would your comments be? Someone who cares for herself and hence takes care – or someone totally disinterested in self and hence in life itself? Dishevelled hair, random application of cosmetics, obese, sloppily dressed, disillusioned and depressed posture? Someone you would like to know, or would sooner forget?

If you like what you see, then you doubtless have a zest for life, are someone good to be with, and are living a satisfactory life. If you are not pleased with the image, then it is time for something to be done before you damage yourself irreversibly. Read on.

2. Imagine yourself as you would like to be

You were not satisfied with the full-length reflection? Then visualize yourself as you would like to be. Consider the points at fault. Think how hair, cosmetics, posture, body weight, dress and so on can be corrected. Imagine your appearance if you did no more than take these simple factors into account and corrected them with a little tender loving care.

Then imagine a little more. New style of dress, slimmer and trimmer, confident upright posture, a smile and not a frown. Do you prefer the new image? Then that must be your objective.

3. Use your tools

The tools available to help you meet your goal have been listed. Use everyone to your advantage. BUT START TODAY.

4. Develop a positive attitude

Consider you yourself first. Remember that you are important and wanted and needed. Decide to live each day to the full. Plan ahead. Become motivated and enthusiastic about yourself, your family and your friends. Enthusiasm is contagious. You will be amazed how your new positive attitude affects your friends and family in a favourable way.

5. Warn your man

The man in your life may well need to look to his laurels himself. In any event, lest he become confused and misinterpret your actions, warn him that today is the first day of the rest of his life and yours. Tell him that you and he are both going places, and along the way are going to enjoy and savour every day and experience to the full.

6. Play the role

Whatever image you have decided you prefer for yourself, must become the role you are going to play. If it is to be a jet-set socialite or a senior tennis champion, the life and fun of the party or a long-distance walker, play the role. This is not a suggestion to mislead yourself or your friends. The recommendation is to have a solid self-image and to live towards fulfilling that image. Above all, try to make your objectives a reality.

7. Get involved

Decide your place within your immediate family circle, your role in the community and your future in society. Be thankful for what you have and what you can expect. More than a third of your life lies ahead of you. Your children are independent, your husband in full career, and for the first time in years you may have spare time on your hands.

Use the time given to you wisely. If you are politically inclined, look towards local government or seek election to Congress. If charitable work attracts you, then find a worthy cause and give of yourself.

Perhaps you once had technical or professional training, only to see your career interrupted by raising a family? Return to University, take a refresher course, go back to work. The pride in fulfilment, the independence of your own salary, the joy of being essential, all these are factors that will boost your self image.

You prefer social activities? Learn to play bridge, join the tennis club, play bowls, start a modern dance group.

The arts is your thing? Take lessons. Keep busy. Plan an exhibition.

And what about the garden? Develop a backyard that will be the envy of your neighbours. Grow the biggest pumpkin.

I am trying to tell you that what you do does not matter. You must enjoy it. Above everything else, GET INVOLVED.

8. Get up and go

This is the final entreaty. And my best wishes for good luck and a happy life go with you.

Appendix I
The Groote Schuur Hospital weight reducing diet

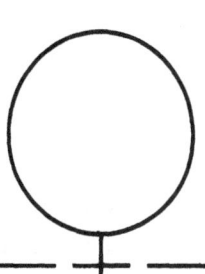

Simple but remarkably effective

The details of this diet are self-explanatory. You limit yourself strictly to the items and amounts of food listed under each meal. For variety you look to the exchange list and swap equivalent items.

Go to it, and keep to it. The results will make the sacrifice worthwhile.

Calories

1000 Calories (4200 Joules) The diet as presented. This is generally recommended.

800 Calories (3300 Joules) Omit two carbohydrate (starch) and one fruit exchange.

600 Calories (2500 Joules) Omit all starch, two fruit exchanges, and butter or other spread.

Daily menu

Breakfast
1 Portion of fruit from exchange list
1 Egg or fish (average helping)
Tomato if desired
1 Portion of starch from exchange list
Tea or coffee with milk from ration

Mid-morning Tea or coffee with milk from ration

Lunch Average portion of lean meat (75 grams), Poultry (75 grams), Fish (120 grams) or skimmed-milk cheese (50 grams)
Vegetables and salads
1 Portion of starch from exchange list
1 Portion of fruit from exchange list
Tea or coffee with milk from ration

Mid-afternoon Tea or coffee with milk from ration
Dinner   Average portion of lean meat, poultry, fish or
                skimmed-milk cheese
                Vegetables and salads
                1 Portion of starch from exchange list
                1 Portion of fruit from exchange list
                Tea or coffee with milk from ration

Daily ration

1/4 litre skimmed milk, fresh or powdered
10 grams (two level teaspoons) of spread (preferably margerine)

Notes

Soda pops and minerals are forbidden.
No sugar allowed in tea or coffee. Use saccharin where available.
Food should be boiled, stewed, steamed or grilled, but not fried.

Exchange list

Carbohydrates (starch)
The following foods are interchangeable. Each amount listed is one
portion of starch.
1 thin slice bread (1 cm thick) 30 grams (equals 1 ounce)
2 medium size potatoes
2 tablespoons rice, macaroni or spaghetti
3 tablespoons beans or peas or sweet potatoes
3 tablespoons cereal
3 crackers
4 Salticrax or water biscuits
2 tablespoons low calorie ice cream
2 level teaspoons cocoa
1 tablespoon nuts.

Fruit
The following fruits are interchangeable. Each amount as listed is
one portion of fruit. They may be raw, stewed or baked.

1 Orange	12 Grapes
1 Apple	½ Cup fresh fruit salad
1 Pear	2 Thin slices pineapple
1 Banana	1 Large slice melon

2 Guavas	1 Large slice watermelon
2 Peaches	6 Prunes
2 Apricots	

Eat as much as you like of the following

Asparagus, cabbage, cauliflower, celery, carrots, cucumber, green beans, leeks, lettuce, marrow, mushrooms, olives, onions, pumpkin, radishes, spinach, squash, tomatoes, turnips, unsweetened pickles. Clear soup, meat and vegetable extracts, soda water, vinegar, pepper, spices.

The following must be omitted

Sugar, glucose, jam, honey, syrup, sweets, chocolates and candy, flour, cakes, sweet biscuits, pastries, puddings, cookies, sweetened canned fruits, oils, fats, sausages and fried foods, beer, stout, sweet wines.

Appendix II
Glossary

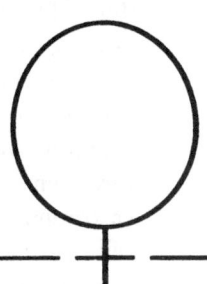

Brief definitions of tongue-twisters

acute sudden onset; opposite of chronic
administer to give treatment
alleviate make less, improve or cure
amenorrhea disappearance of menstrual periods
anatomy description of body parts or structures
androgens hormones with male-like effects
anus the opening of the lower bowel to the outside
anxiety worrying without having something to worry about
atheromatosis fatty disease of the blood vessels
artery the blood vessels that leave the heart for the rest of the
body
atrophic vaginitis thinning and inflammation of the vagina
Bartholin's gland two glands at the entrance of the vagina that
respond to sexual arousal by producing lubricating mucus
birth control pill the oral contraceptive; combination of estrogen
and progestin in a pill which prevents ovulation and pregnancy.
bladder the storage bag in which urine collects before release
blood clot a congealed lump of blood inside the blood vessel
blood stream the rivers of blood inside the blood vessels
blood vessels the tubes called arteries or veins in which blood
flows
brain the grey lump of nervous tissue inside the skull
breakthrough bleeding vaginal bleeding that actually starts whilst
taking female hormones or oral contraceptives
breast milk producing gland
calcium the major chemical substance needed to harden bones
and teeth

calories essentially a measure of how much energy is present in the food that you eat

cancer uncontrolled growth of abnormal tissue which spreads and destroys normal tissue

carcinoma see *cancer*

castration removal of a woman's ovaries or a man's testicles

cell the basic unit or building block out of which all body tissues are constructed

cervix the mouth of the womb; the entrance of the uterus

change of life see *climacteric*

chronic present or developing over a long time. Opposite of acute

climacteric the transition from reproductive to postreproductive age

climacteric syndrome symptoms associated with climacteric

clitoris a small structure near the entrance of the vulva that is responsive to sexual stimulation

complaint a symptom bad enough to bother you and to report to the doctor

complication an adverse effect; development of one disease on another

compression fracture a weakened bone cannot support weight and can break by being crushed

contraindication circumstances in which a drug should not be prescribed

coronary artery disease fatty disease of the arteries of the heart can lead to plugging with a blood clot; see atheromatosis

corpus luteum the yellow body in the ovary that forms from the graafian follicle after ovulation

culture the usual beliefs, social behaviour and material components of a racial, religious or social group, normally passed from one generation to the next

cycle a recurring series of events; moving in a circle

cyclical used to refer to medical treatment of a regular but recurring on-off-on schedule

D. and C. (dilatation and curettage) common gynaecologic operation in which the cervix is opened or stretched (dilatation), and the lining of the uterus is scraped with an instrument called a curette

deficiency disease certain substances necessary to the body may be absent or in short supply and this leads to disease

degeneration decay

diabetes deficiency disease due to lack of insulin

diuretic water-losing pill

dosage the actual amount of the drug to be given or taken

drug a medication, but not necessarily an addictive substance

dyspareunia the development of pain related to sexual intercourse

ERT Estrogen Replacement Therapy; the popular term used for long-term estrogen treatment

edema accumulation of fluid in the body with swelling

embryo the early structure resulting from fertilization of sperm and egg

endocrine gland specialized body gland that produces hormones

endometrium the lining of the uterus

environment conditions, objects and circumstances that surround one

estrogen the female sex hormone which is produced by the ovaries

FSH (follicle stimulating hormone) a hormone secreted by the pituitary gland that stimulates the follicle in the ovary to grow

fallacy false idea

fallopian tube tube from uterus which opens near ovary and acts as duct for sperm and egg

fertile to be able to have a baby

fertilization the joining of the egg and sperm

fetus the baby growing inside the uterus before birth

flashes see *hot flushes*

fluid retention see *edema*

fracture the breaking of a bone

genital atrophy the shrivelling or wasting away of the female organs

genitals the female or male sex organs

gland body structure that secretes fluid or chemicals

GRH (gonadotropin releasing hormone) the hormone made by the hypothalamus that stimulates the pituitary gland to produce gonadotropins

gonad sex organ containing sperm or eggs; testicle in the male and ovary in the female

gonadotropin a hormone that can stimulate the gonad and produced by the pituitary

hormone   chemical messenger produced by the endocrine gland
HRT   similar to ERT
hot flushes   feeling of heat that spreads over arms, chest and face
hypertension   high blood pressure
hysterectomy   removal of the uterus at surgery
hypothalamus   the co-ordinating centre of the brain which lies above the pituitary gland
implant   hard lump of hormone placed in the body fat under the skin, usually of estrogen and inserted every couple of months
insomnia   inability to get to sleep
jaundice   yellow colour of the skin and eyes, usually due to liver disease
LH (luteinizing hormone)   the pituitary hormone which stimulates release of the egg from the graafian follicle and formation of the corpus luteum
labia majora   the outer lips of the entrance to the vagina
labia minora   the inner lips of the entrance to the vagina
laparotomy   opening of the abdominal cavity surgically to explore the interior
menarche   the first menstrual period
menopause   the final menstrual period
menstrual flow   the period or monthly flow of blood from the vagina
menstrual irregularity   vaginal bleeding at abnormal or irregular times
menstrual period   the monthly flow of vaginal bleeding indicating no pregnancy has occurred
menstruation   the monthly period
mortality rate   number of deaths occurring per certain total population
natural estrogens   estrogens similar to ones made normally by the body
nausea   desire to vomit
obese   extremely fat
oophorectomy   the removal of one or both ovaries at surgery
orgasm   the sexual climax
osteoporosis   thinning of bone
ovariectomy   see *oophorectomy*
ovary   the female organ containing eggs and making sex hormones

ovulation escape of the egg from the graafian follicle of the ovary

PAP smear scraping from the cervix to detect early cancerous changes

pathology science of the study of disease in organs

pelvis bony basin around the lower abdominal organs

perimenopause the time around menopause; see *climacteric*

period see *menstruation*

pharmaceutical company company which makes medications

pharmacology science of the study of drugs

physiology science of the study of function of the body

pituitary gland an endocrine gland in the skull

postmenopause after the menopause

postmenopausal syndrome see *climacteric syndrome*

potent extremely powerful

primordial follicle the early follicle in the ovary made up of the egg surrounded by cells

progesterone one of the ovarian female hormones, it controls the action of estrogen

progestin synthetic drugs with structure and effect like progesterone

prolapse sagging or dropping of uterus, bladder and vagina due to loss of pelvic support

psychogenic problem caused by a mental rather than a physical disturbance

psychology science of the study of behaviour

puberty transition from childhood to reproductive age

pubic hair the hair on the external genitals

ratio numerical comparison between one thing and another, for example, risk to benefit

regime plan for a course of treatment

reproductive organs ovaries, fallopian tubes, uterus and vagina

secrete production and release of a substance from a gland

sexual intercourse the act of making love

side effect an undesirable reaction produced by a drug

social relates to the structure and way of thinking of a community

spotting irregular, slight vaginal bleeding between periods

stress incontinence inability to hold urine in properly during coughing, laughing or sneezing

surgical menopause menopause following surgical removal of the ovaries

syndrome a set of symptoms put together as a group

symptom the feeling which alerts the body about something wrong

synthetic estrogens estrogens made artificially in a laboratory

testes the testicle or gland in the male that produces sperm

testosterone the male hormone made by the testes

therapy treatment

thromboembolism breaking off of blood clot in one part of the body and its travelling to another part via the bloodstream

urethra the tube from the bladder through which urine escapes

uterus the womb

vagina muscular tube for sex; also the birth canal

vaginal smear vaginal wall scraping for laboratory testing

vein blood vessels carrying blood from the body to the heart

vulva the outside of the female genitalia

womb the uterus

Appendix III
Further reading

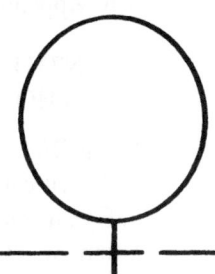

Hopefully no longer necessary at this stage

General

Ageing and estrogens   Frontiers of Hormone Research, Vol. 2. Editors: P. A. van Keep and C. Lauritzen. Karger, Basle, 1973.

Consensus on Menopause Research   A Summary of International Opinion. Editors: P. A. van Keep, R. B. Greenblatt, M. Albeaux-Fernet MTP Press, Lancaster, 1976.

Estrogens in the postmenopause   Frontiers of Hormone Research, Vol. 3. Editors: P. A. van Keep and C. Lauritzen. Karger, Basle, 1975.

Menstruation and menopause   Paula Weideger. Knopf, New York, 1976.

Oestrogen therapy during the climacteric and afterwards   P. A. van Keep and A. A. Haspels. Excerpta Medica, Amsterdam, 1977.

Our bodies, our selves   Boston Women's Health Collective. Simon and Schuster, New York, 1973.

Physical fitness   XBX 12-minute-a-day Plan for Women. Royal Canadian Air Force. Penguin Books, Harmondsworth, 1960.

Sex and the life cycle   Editors: W. A. Oaks, G. A. Melchiode and I. Ficher. Grune and Stratton, New York, 1976.

The AMA book of skin and hair care   Editor: Linda Allen Schoen. J. B. Lippincott Co., New York, 1974.

The menopause   A Guide to Current Research and Practice. Editor: R. J. Beard. MTP Press, Lancaster, 1976.

SCIENTIFIC PUBLICATIONS ON MENOPAUSE BY THE AUTHOR

Utian, W. H. Feminine Forever? Current concepts on the menopause. A critical review. *South African Journal of Obstetrics and Gynaecology*, **6**, 7–10, 1968.

Utian, W. H. The pros and cons of long-term oestrogen administration to the postmenopausal female. *Medical Proceedings*, **15**, 307–313, 1969.

Utian, W. H. and Adler, M. Chronic low backache in the middle-aged woman. *South African Journal of Physiotherapy*, **22**, 5–8, 1970.

Utian, W. H. Clinical and metabolic effects of the menopause and the role of replacement oestrogen therapy. *Thesis, Doctor of Philosophy, University of Cape Town*, 1970.

Utian, W. H. Use of vaginal smear in assessment of oestrogenic status of oophorectomised females. *South African Journal of Obstetrics and Gynaecology*, **8**, 69–72, 1970.

Utian, W. H. Cholesterol, coronary heart disease and oestrogens. *South African Medical Journal*, **45**, 359, 1971.

Utian, W. H. Oestrogens and osteoporosis. *South African Medical Journal*, **45**, 879–882, 1971.

Utian, W. H. Effects of oophorectomy and estrogen therapy on serum cholesterol. *International Journal of Obstetrics and Gynecology*, **10**, 95–101, 1972.

Utian, W. H. The true clinical features of postmenopause and oophorectomy, and their response to oestrogen therapy. *South African Medical Journal*, **46**, 732–737, 1972.

Utian, W. H. Effects of oophorectomy and subsequent oestrogen therapy on plasma calcium and phosphorus. *South African Journal of Obstetrics and Gynaecology*, **10**, 8–16, 1972.

Utian, W. H. The mental tonic effect of oestrogens administered to oophorectomised females. *South African Medical Journal* **46**, 1079–1082, 1972.

Utian, W. H. Comparative trial of P1496, a new non-steroidal oestrogen analogue. *British Medical Journal*, **1**, 579–581, 1973.

George, G. C. W., Utian, W. H., Beumont, P. J. V., and Beardwood, C. J. Effect of exogenous oestrogen on minor psychiatric symptoms in postmenopausal women. *South African Medical Journal*,

47, 2387–2388, 1973.

Utian, W. H. Oestrogen, headache and oral contraceptives. *South African Medical Journal*, **48**, 2105–2108, 1974.

Utian, W. H. Osteoporosis, oestrogens and oophorectomy. A proposed new test of oestrogenic potency. *South African Medical Journal*, **49**, 433–436, 1975.

Utian, W. H., Vinik, A. I., Beardwood, C. J. and Beumont, P. V. J. Effect of Congjugated Oestrogen therapy on circulating luteinising hormone in oophorectomised women. *South African Medical Journal*, **49**, 821–822, 1975.

Utian, W. H. Definitive symptoms of postmenopause – incorporating use of vaginal parabasal cell index. Estrogens in the postmenopause, *Frontiers of Hormone Research*, **3**, 74–93, Karger, Basle, 1975.

Utian, W. H. Effect of hysterectomy, oophorectomy and estrogen therapy on libido. *International Journal of Gynecology and Obstetrics*, **13**, 97–100, 1975.

Utian, W. H. Mental tonic effect of estrogen therapy in postmenopause. In: *The Family. Proceedings of the Fourth International Congress of Psychosomatic Obstetrics and Gynecology.* Karger, Basle, 1975.

Utian, W. H. The scientific basis for postmenopausal estrogen therapy: The management of specific symptoms and rationale for long-term replacement. In: *The Menopause, A Guide to Current Research and Practice.* MTP Press, Lancaster, 1976.

Utian, W. H. Effect of hysterectomy, oophorectomy and estrogen therapy on libido. *Obstetrical and Gynecological Survey*, **31**, 319–321, 1976.

Utian, W. H., and Serr, D. the climacteric syndrome. In: *Consensus on Menopause Research.* Editors: P. A. van Keep, R. B. Greenblatt and M. Albeaux-Fernet. MTP Press, Lancaster, 1976.

Utian, W. H. Current status of menopause and postmenopausal estrogen therapy. *Obstetrical and Gynecological Survey*, **32**, 193–204, 1977.

Utian, W. H. The menopause and its management – the risk : cost : benefit ratio. *South African Journal of Hospital Medicine*, **3**, 304–307, 1977.

Utian, W. H. Effect of postmenopausal estrogen therapy on diastolic blood pressure and body weight. *Maturitas* **1**, 3–8, 1978.

Utian, W. H., Katz, M., Davey, D. and Carr, P. J. Effect of premenopausal castration and incremental dosages of conjugated equine estrogens on plasma FSH, LH and estradiol. *American Journal of Obstetrics and Gynecology* (In press), 1978.

Index